Fast Facts

Fast Facts:
Renal Disorders

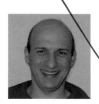

Jeremy Levy MA PhD ILTM FRCP
Consultant Nephrologist
Hammersmith Hospitals NHS Trust
London, UK

Charles Pusey DSc FRCP FRCPath FMedSci
Professor of Medicine
Head of Department of Renal Medicine
Imperial College London
London, UK

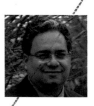

Ajay Singh MD
Associate Professor of Medicine, Harvard Medical School
Clinical Director of the Renal Division
Brigham and Women's Hospital
Boston, MA, USA

Declaration of Independence
This book is as balanced and as practical as
we can make it. Ideas for improvement are
always welcome: feedback@fastfacts.com

HEALTH PRESS

Fast Facts: Renal Disorders
First published February 2006

Health Press Limited, Elizabeth House, Queen Street, Abingdon,
Oxford OX14 3LN, UK
Tel: +44 (0)1235 523233
Fax: +44 (0)1235 523238

Book orders can be placed by telephone or via the website.
For regional distributors or to order via the website, please go to:
www.fastfacts.com
For telephone orders, please call 01752 202301 (UK), +44 1752 202301 (Europe),
1 800 247 6553 (USA, toll free) or +1 419 281 1802 (Americas).

Fast Facts is a trademark of Health Press Limited.

Medical illustrations by Dee McLean, London, UK.
Typesetting and page layout by Zed, Oxford, UK.
Printed by Fine Print (Services) Ltd, Oxford, UK.

Printed with vegetable inks on fully biodegradable and
recyclable paper manufactured from sustainable forests.

444   001
Low emissions
during production

Low
chlorine

Sustainable
forests

Glossary of abbreviations   4

Introduction   5

Proteinuria, hematuria and renal investigations   7

Electrolyte disturbances and acid–base disorders   17

Acute renal failure   33

Chronic kidney disease   41

Hypertension and diabetic nephropathy   58

Glomerulonephritis   74

Systemic disease   83

Inherited kidney diseases   92

Urinary tract infections   98

Kidney stones   108

Urinary tract obstruction and tumors   118

Pregnancy and renal disease   128

Renal replacement therapy and renal transplantation   133

Useful addresses   144

Index   146

Glossary of abbreviations

ACE: angiotensin-converting enzyme

ADH: antidiuretic hormone

AKPD: autosomal-dominant polycystic kidney disease

ANCA: antineutrophil cytoplasm antibody

ARB: angiotensin-receptor blocker

ARF: acute renal failure

ATN: acute tubular necrosis

BPH: benign prostatic hyperplasia

BUN: blood urea nitrogen (also known as serum urea)

cANCA: cytoplasmic antineutrophil cytoplasm antibody

CKD: chronic kidney disease

CT: computerized tomography

ECG: electrocardiogram

ESR: erythrocyte sedimentation rate

ESRF: end-stage renal failure

ESWL: extracorporeal shock-wave lithotripsy

GFR: glomerular filtration rate

HIV: human immunodeficiency virus

HUS: hemolytic uremic syndrome

Ig: immunoglobulin

LDL: low-density lipoprotein

MCGN: mesangiocapillary glomerulonephritis

MDRD: modification of diet in renal disease

NSAIDs: non-steroidal anti-inflammatory drugs

pANCA: perinuclear antineutrophil cytoplasm antibody

PTH: parathyroid hormone

SIADH: syndrome of inappropriate secretion of ADH

SLE: systemic lupus erythematosus

TTP: thrombotic thrombocytopenic purpura

UTI: urinary tract infection

Introduction

Kidney disease is common and its prevalence is increasing worldwide. Up to 8% of the population of developed countries have some degree of renal impairment; in the USA, over 19 million adults have some form of chronic kidney disease (CKD) and 1 in 1000 is receiving treatment for end-stage renal failure (ESRF). It is estimated that the direct medical costs of ESRF exceed US$15 billion per year in the USA; the total cost of dialysis is over US$77 000/patient/year in the UK.

CKD is often a progressive condition, but the rate of decline can be slowed and complications can be substantially reduced by timely treatment. This is especially important for the increasing number of patients with diabetes and hypertension in whom treatment can greatly reduce renal morbidity (see Chapter 5).

Acute renal failure is significantly less common, but still affects 5% of hospitalized patients. Although it is an important cause of morbidity and mortality, it can often be treated successfully.

It is therefore important for all physicians, both in hospitals and the community, to have an awareness of renal disease, its management and its complications. We hope this book will help to achieve this.

Proteinuria, hematuria and renal investigations

The clinical symptoms of renal disease often do not become apparent until renal failure is advanced. Screening for renal disease is, therefore, particularly important, because it may enable abnormalities to be detected in time for effective treatment to be started. Bedside urine analysis is an essential part of any clinical examination. Urine testing may also be part of a routine medical examination for insurance or employment purposes, or when a person registers with a new primary care physician.

Urinary abnormalities will be found in most patients with renal disease, particularly positive dipstick tests for blood or protein, or the presence of cells, casts, crystals or organisms on urine microscopy. Clinically, severe hematuria may be reported if the patient has red or dark urine, which, if it occurs at the end of the urinary stream, suggests bleeding from the lower urinary tract. Heavy proteinuria can produce unusually frothy urine, but this is not often reported spontaneously.

Proteinuria

Proteinuria may originate from anywhere within the urinary tract. High protein levels generally reflect glomerular disease (glomerular proteinuria), and albumin is the main component. Proteinuria occurring as a result of tubular damage is usually only low level and involves proteins of a lower molecular weight, such as β_2-microglobulin. Overflow proteinuria may occur as a result of the filtration of abnormal amounts of low-molecular-weight proteins through the glomeruli, such as monoclonal light chains in myeloma. One of the most common causes of low-level proteinuria is inflammation in the lower urinary tract, which is usually caused by urinary infection (Table 1.1).

Dipstick testing of the urine is designed to detect albumin and is insensitive to other proteins; it will not, therefore, generally detect light chains in myeloma. Dipsticks may detect albumin in concentrations as

TABLE 1.1

Causes of proteinuria

Glomerular proteinuria (most common cause)
- Primary glomerulonephritis of all histological types
- Secondary glomerular disease due to diabetes, systemic lupus erythematosus or amyloidosis

Tubular proteinuria
- Tubulointerstitial nephritis, often related to drugs, but with many other causes
- Toxins damaging the tubule, such as heavy metals and tetracycline

Overflow proteinuria
- Multiple myeloma and monoclonal immunoglobulin deposition disease
- Myoglobinuria
- Hemoglobinuria

Tissue proteinuria
- Acute inflammation of urinary tract
- Urinary tract tumors

low as 20–30 mg/dL, and are often calibrated on a scale of 0–3+, which provides a semiquantitative estimate of protein concentration. False-positive results may occur if the urine is highly concentrated, and false-negative results if the urine is very dilute.

Proteinuria may be formally quantified using timed urine samples, usually a 24-hour specimen. The upper end of the normal range is taken as 200 mg/24 hours. As collecting 24-hour urine samples is difficult and unreliable, measurement of the protein:creatinine ratio using a spot urine sample is increasingly being used, because it correlates well with 24-hour protein excretion. In conventional units a protein:creatinine ratio of 1 equates to 1 g/24 hours protein excretion, and in SI units a ratio of 120 mg/mmol equates to 1 g/24 hours proteinuria. Proteinuria of more than 1 g/24 hours, in the absence of an obvious cause, should prompt further investigation, which often includes renal biopsy. Proteinuria of more than 3.5 g/24 hours commonly leads to nephrotic syndrome (see Chapter 5).

Hematuria

Whereas significant proteinuria often indicates intrinsic renal disease, hematuria is commonly caused by lesions throughout the urinary tract, particularly infection or malignancy (Table 1.2).

Dipstick testing of the urine provides a semiquantitative estimate of the degree of hematuria, but hemoglobin (in hemolysis) and myoglobin (in rhabdomyolysis) may produce positive tests. Urine microscopy should always be performed to detect red blood cells. Misshapen or dysmorphic red cells, detected by an experienced observer using phase-contrast microscopy, suggest glomerular hematuria. The presence of red-cell or granular casts in the urine is a more reliable way of identifying a renal source of the hematuria, as opposed to a ureteric or bladder source. Red-cell casts, in particular, generally indicate active glomerulonephritis. In most cases, significant proteinuria in addition to hematuria is seen in glomerular disease. Several clinical algorithms have been proposed for the investigation of hematuria (Figure 1.1). In general, once urinary tract infection has been excluded, then hematuria *without* significant proteinuria should prompt a search for malignancy in older patients, while hematuria with proteinuria requires a search for a glomerular cause.

Renal function tests

Renal function is assessed most simply by measuring the concentrations of metabolites excreted by the kidney, the most commonly used metabolites being urea and creatinine. The urea concentration is influenced more by dietary intake of protein, the state of hydration, liver function and various drugs. Serum creatinine is, therefore, a more reliable measure, but is related directly to muscle mass; thus, a small elderly woman may have a normal serum creatinine with a markedly reduced glomerular filtration rate (GFR). Changes in serum creatinine (especially a rise) can be a useful guide to deteriorating renal function; absolute values do not correlate well with GFR. Creatinine clearance, which assesses creatinine excretion over 24 hours in relation to the

TABLE 1.2

Causes of hematuria

Glomerular disease

- Most types of primary glomerulonephritis (rare in membranous and minimal change disease)
- Secondary glomerulonephritis due to systemic vasculitis, systemic lupus erythematosus, Goodpasture's syndrome, Henoch–Schönlein purpura or postinfectious nephritis
- Hereditary nephritis, such as Alport's syndrome and thin basement membrane disease

Disease of the interstitium or tubule

- Acute interstitial nephritis, particularly due to drugs
- Hereditary disease, such as polycystic kidney disease and medullary sponge kidney
- Vascular disorders, such as malignant hypertension and renal artery embolism (including cholesterol emboli)
- Papillary necrosis due to diabetes, sickle-cell disease and analgesic abuse

Disease of the renal pelvis, ureter and bladder

- Transitional cell carcinoma
- Bladder carcinoma
- Calculi
- Infection (e.g. tuberculosis, schistosomiasis)
- Acute inflammation (e.g. urinary tract infection)
- Toxins (e.g. cyclophosphamide)
- Trauma

Coagulation disturbances

- Abnormalities of the coagulation system or platelets (many inherited and acquired disorders)

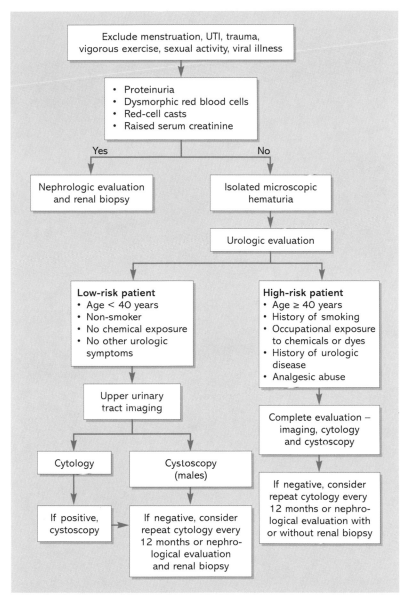

Figure 1.1 An algorithm for the investigation of hematuria.

serum creatinine level, is often used as a measure of GFR. However, it can overestimate GFR, since up to 25% of urinary creatinine may come from tubular secretion, and 24-hour urine collections are unreliable.

It is also important to realize that a significant rise in serum creatinine does not occur until the GFR is reduced to about 50% of normal.

A number of formulas have been described to estimate GFR based on the serum creatinine and the characteristics of the patient (e.g. age, weight, sex, race). The two best-known formulas are the Cockcroft–Gault and the Modification of Diet in Renal Disease study (MDRD) formulas (Table 1.3). The MDRD is more accurate, but is rather more complicated. Newer methods, which may find their way into clinical practice, include iohexol clearance and serum cystatin concentration.

TABLE 1.3

Formulas for calculating creatinine clearance or glomerular filtration rate

Cockcroft–Gault formula (SI units)

$(140 - \text{age}) \times \text{weight (kg)} / \text{serum creatinine (μmol/L)} \times 1.23$ if male or $\times 1.04$ if female

Cockcroft–Gault (conventional units)

$[(140 - \text{age}) \times \text{weight (kg)} / \text{serum creatinine (mg/dL)} \times 72]$ if male $\times 0.85$ if female

MDRD formula (SI units)

$170 \times (\text{serum creatinine [μmol/L]} \times 0.0114)^{-0.999} \times \text{age}^{-0.176} \times (\text{blood urea nitrogen [serum urea]} \times 2.8)^{-0.17} \times \text{albumin}^{0.318} \times 0.762$ if female $\times 1.18$ if black

MDRD formula (conventional units)

$170 \times \text{serum creatinine (mg/dL)}^{-0.999} \times \text{age}^{-0.176} \times (\text{blood urea nitrogen [serum urea]})^{-0.17} \times \text{albumin}^{0.318} \times 0.762$ if female $\times 1.18$ if black

MDRD formula – brief version (SI units)

$186 \times (\text{serum creatinine [mmol/L]} \times 0.0114)^{-1.154} \times \text{age}^{-0.203} \times 0.742$ if female $\times 1.21$ if black

MDRD formula – brief version (conventional units)

$186 \times \text{serum creatinine (mg/dL)}^{-1.154} \times \text{age}^{-0.203} \times 0.742$ if female $\times 1.21$ if black

Other blood tests

The diagnosis of many renal diseases is assisted by specific blood tests, particularly in glomerular disease. These tests include measurement of blood glucose for diabetes mellitus, and serum electrophoresis for myeloma and other B-cell dyscrasias. A range of immunological tests (e.g. anti-DNA antibodies and complement levels in systemic lupus erythematosus [SLE]; see Chapter 4) is helpful in the diagnosis of glomerulonephritis.

Renal imaging

The investigation of renal disease should always include some form of renal imaging, which can provide both anatomic and functional information (Figure 1.2 and Table 1.4). In general, it is appropriate to start with cheaper, non-invasive methods of imaging, such as ultrasonography, and use more invasive and expensive methods selectively.

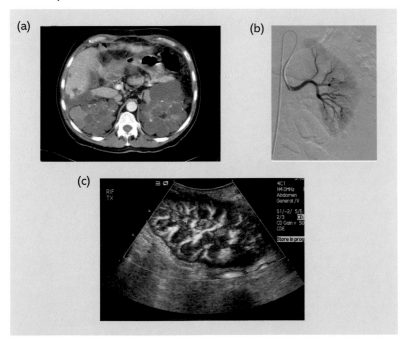

Figure 1.2 Renal investigations: (a) a CT scan; (b) an angiogram and (c) an ultrasound scan.

TABLE 1.4

Renal imaging techniques

Indication	Major advantages
Ultrasonography	
• Estimate kidney size (differentiate acute from chronic kidney disease) • Detect structural abnormalities (e.g. cysts, reflux) • Exclude obstruction • Guide biopsy or nephrostomy	• Cheap • Easy to perform • Portable
Doppler ultrasonography	
• Screen for renal artery stenosis or thrombosis	• Cheap • Reliable if good Doppler signals obtained
Computerized tomography	
• Provide detailed anatomic information about the kidneys • Examine ureters and bladder	• Good anatomic detail
Magnetic resonance imaging	
• Provide anatomic information about the kidneys • Examine ureters and bladder • Define renovascular lesions	• Nephrotoxic contrast not used
Radionucleotide imaging	
• Provide functional information about each kidney • Screen for renovascular disease (with captopril) or obstruction (with furosemide) • Obtain quantitative functional data	• Nephrotoxic contrast not used
Renal angiography	
• Gold standard for detection of renovascular disorders including renal artery stenosis and aneurysms • Provide intervention for angioplasty, stenting or embolization	• Excellent definition of vascular anatomy and opportunity for intervention

> **Key points – proteinuria, hematuria and renal investigations**
>
> • Proteinuria and hematuria should always be investigated.
> • Proteinuria should be quantified by means of protein:creatinine ratios or 24-hour collections, since the result will guide management.
> • Hematuria may have a medical or surgical cause, and this should be assessed before starting investigations.
> • Serum creatinine alone is an unreliable guide to renal function; an assessment of glomerular filtration rate is more useful.

Renal biopsy

Percutaneous renal biopsy can provide a definitive histological diagnosis of glomerular or interstitial disease. It is particularly helpful in patients with severe proteinuria, hematuria that is not due to disease of the lower urinary tract, and acute renal failure thought to be caused by intrinsic renal disease (rather than prerenal disease, obstruction or acute tubular necrosis [ATN]). The main diseases diagnosed by renal biopsy include glomerulonephritis, glomerular disorders such as amyloid and diabetes, and interstitial nephritis. Opinions differ as to when renal biopsy is indicated, but the potential benefit in terms of treatment should outweigh the risk involved (significant bleeding in about 1 in 1000 cases). If both kidneys are small, as in chronic glomerulonephritis, then the risk generally outweighs the benefit. In the presence of microscopic hematuria alone, or proteinuria of less than 1 g/24 hours, renal biopsy is often not indicated since it is unlikely that a specific treatment would be required. However, higher levels of proteinuria, or the combination of proteinuria and hematuria (particularly with casts) are indications for biopsy, because a number of causes of glomerulonephritis (see Chapter 6) and interstitial nephritis are now amenable to therapy.

Key references

Khadra MH, Pickard RS, Charlton M et al. A prospective analysis of 1,930 patients with hematuria to evaluate current diagnostic practice. *J Urol* 2000;163:524–7.

Johnson CA, Levey AS, Coresh J et al. Clinical practice guidelines for chronic kidney disease in adults: Part II. Glomerular filtration rate, proteinuria, and other markers. *Am Fam Physician* 2004;70:1091–7.

Rockall AJ, Newman-Sanders AP, al-Kutoubi MA, Vale JA. Haematuria. *Postgrad Med J* 1997;73:129–36.

2 Electrolyte disturbances and acid–base disorders

Plasma electrolyte and acid–base disturbances are common clinical problems. Perturbations may result in morbidity and mortality, particularly in the elderly and young children, and in those with other comorbid states, such as sepsis, coronary heart disease and heart failure.

Sodium and water disorders

Regulation of the plasma sodium concentration by the body relies on the balance of intake and excretion of both sodium and water, and the function of sensors of osmolality and extracellular fluid volume, such as hypothalamic osmoreceptors and carotid baroreceptors, and effector mechanisms such as antidiuretic hormone (ADH) and aldosterone.

Hyponatremia. Mild hyponatremia (plasma sodium 130–135 mmol/L) is common and affects approximately 15–20% of hospitalized patients. More severe hyponatremia (plasma sodium < 130 mmol/L) is rarer and occurs in less than 1–4% of patients (Table 2.1).

Clinical features. Hyponatremia in conjunction with hypo-osmolality (as is common) causes clinical problems, especially when the plasma sodium concentration falls below 120 mmol/L, and patients usually complain of nausea and malaise. When the plasma sodium reaches 115 mmol/L, patients may complain of headache and become delirious. Seizures and coma are common when the plasma sodium falls below 110 mmol/L. These neurological complications reflect water shifting osmotically into the brain. Premenopausal women and children seem to be particularly susceptible to symptomatic hyponatremia for reasons that are unclear.

Diagnosis of hypo-osmolar hyponatremia requires careful assessment of extracellular volume and measurement of urinary sodium to determine whether total body sodium is low, normal or high. Adrenal failure, renal failure and hypothyroidism must always be excluded.

TABLE 2.1

Causes of hyponatremia and hypo-osmolality

Hypovolemic hyponatremia (reduction in total body sodium)

- Renal losses – diuretics, hypoaldosteronism, salt wasting nephropathy
- Gastrointestinal – vomiting, diarrhea, enteral tube drainage
- Skin – excessive sweating, burns

Euvolemic hyponatremia (normal total body sodium)

- Syndrome of inappropriate antidiuretic hormone secretion (SIADH)
- Cortisol deficiency
- Renal failure
- Hypothyroidism
- Pregnancy
- Pyschosis
- Primary polydipsia

Hypervolemic hyponatremia (increased total body sodium)

- Heart failure
- Nephrotic syndrome
- Cirrhosis

The history and physical examination should focus on identifying any underlying cause of the hyponatremia, such as a malignancy causing a syndrome of inappropriate secretion of ADH (SIADH). Investigations should confirm hypo-osmolality, and demonstrate either appropriate or inappropriate secretion of ADH by comparing urine osmolality with plasma osmolality. Urine osmolality below 100 mOsmol/kg (i.e. very dilute urine) indicates that ADH secretion is completely and appropriately suppressed. Urine osmolality above 100 mOsmol/kg, and particularly in the range of 200–600 mOsmol/kg, indicates either exogenous appropriate or inappropriate secretion of ADH. A diagnosis of SIADH can be easily made based on specific diagnostic criteria (Tables 2.2 and 2.3).

TABLE 2.2

Common disorders associated with the syndrome of inappropriate antidiuretic hormone secretion (SIADH)

Pulmonary

- Abscess
- Tuberculosis
- Pneumonia
- Aspergillosis
- Positive-pressure ventilation
- Asthma

Neoplastic

- Lung
- Pancreas
- Lymphoma
- Stomach
- Prostate cancer
- Bladder cancer

Neurological

- Neoplasm
- Head trauma
- Encephalitis
- Meningitis
- Brain abscess
- Guillain–Barré syndrome

TABLE 2.3

Diagnostic criteria for syndrome of inappropriate antidiuretic hormone secretion (SIADH)

- Hyponatremia and hypo-osmolality
- Normal extracellular volume
- Urine osmolality > 100 mOsmol/kg
- Urine sodium > 20 mmol/L
- Normal renal, adrenal, hepatic and thyroid function

Treatment. Particular care must be taken when correcting hyponatremia in premenopausal women, children and those with very low plasma sodium levels (< 120 mmol/L). Severe symptomatic

19

hyponatremia may require treatment with hypertonic (3%) sodium chloride. The sodium concentration should be monitored frequently. The optimal correction rate should be 0.5–1 mmol/L/hour, with a total correction of plasma sodium of 10–12 mmol over the first 24 hours. A more aggressive correction rate of 2.0 mmol/L/hour may be considered in patients with seizures or severe neurological symptoms attributable to hyponatremia. However, an overly rapid correction rate carries the risk of precipitating central pontine myelinolysis.

Hypernatremia (plasma sodium concentration ≥ 145 mmol/L) is common among hospitalized patients, particularly the elderly. Hypernatremia is also often seen in individuals who have lost their perception of thirst (e.g. as a result of a neurological disability) or who have been denied free access to water (Table 2.4). Hypernatremia always reflects a state of hyperosmolality. Since sodium is usually confined to the extracellular space, an actual or relative increase in sodium (compared with water) results in the movement of water out of

TABLE 2.4

Causes of hypernatremia and hyperosmolality

Hypovolemic hypernatremia (reduction in total body sodium)

- Skin – burns, excessive sweating
- Gastrointestinal – diarrhea, vomiting

Euvolemic hypernatremia (normal total body sodium)

- Skin – burns, excessive sweating
- Respiratory – tachypnea
- Renal losses
- Central diabetes insipidus
- Nephrogenic diabetes insipidus

Hypervolemic hypernatremia (increased total body sodium)

- Hypertonic parenteral nutrition
- Hypertonic saline or sodium bicarbonate administration

cells driven by osmosis. Cellular dehydration follows, and shrinkage of brain cells causes most of the clinical manifestations.

Clinical features. Mild hypernatremia (plasma sodium 150–155 mmol/L) is usually associated with nausea, vomiting, irritability and a depressed sensorium. More severe hypernatremia (plasma sodium > 160 mmol/L) may result in seizures, focal neurological defects, stupor and coma. In children, muscle spasticity, fever and labored respiration may be prominent.

The speed with which hypernatremia develops also appears to modulate the severity of the clinical features. Severe, acute hypernatremia may result in irreversible vascular damage, particularly among children. Acute hypernatremia is associated with a mortality of 40%, whereas chronic hypernatremia is associated with a mortality of 10%.

Diagnosis. The differential diagnosis of hypernatremia requires an initial assessment of extracellular volume (Figure 2.1). The history and physical examination should focus on identifying any underlying cause.

Treatment. Hypovolemic hypernatremic patients can be managed by administration of isotonic saline. Patients with hypervolemic hypernatremia are treated with diuretics and free water given orally or parenterally (5% dextrose). Euvolemic hypernatremic patients can be treated with free water orally or 5% dextrose infusion. Too rapid correction is associated with brain edema, caused by the rapid movement of water into the brain, and seizures. In most circumstances, a correction rate of about 0.5 mmol/L/hour should suffice.

Potassium disorders

Potassium is predominantly found intracellularly. Excretion of potassium is largely achieved by the kidneys, but also to a lesser extent by the colon. Transcellular shifts of potassium between the intracellular and extracellular compartments also occur.

Hypokalemia (plasma potassium ≤ 3.5 mmol/L) is one of the most common electrolyte abnormalities in hospitalized patients (Table 2.5).

Clinical features largely reflect alterations in membrane polarization, especially in cardiac and skeletal muscle. Changes in the

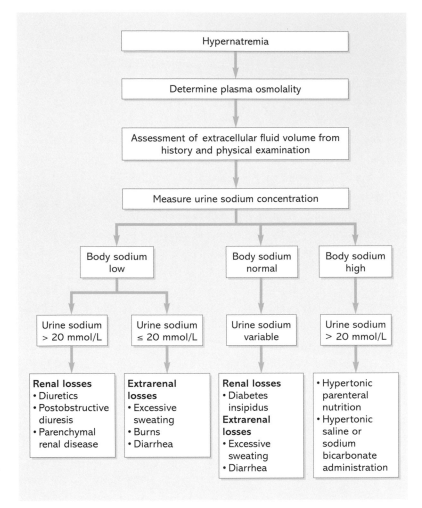

Figure 2.1 Diagnostic approach to the causes of hypernatremia.

electrocardiogram (ECG) include flattening of the T wave, depression of ST segments and a prominent U wave. Hypokalemia also increases predisposition to arrhythmias, particularly in patients with digoxin toxicity or those with acute coronary syndromes. The affects of hypokalemia on skeletal muscle range from weakness, tetany and fatigue to rhabdomyolosis. Severe hypokalemia (plasma potassium < 2.0 mmol/L) can lead to paralysis. Chronic hypokalemia can also cause a reduction in GFR, interstitial scarring and tubular atrophy.

TABLE 2.5

Causes of hypokalemia

Reduced intake
- Dietary deficiency (tea-and-toast diet)

Transcellular shifts
- Catecholamines (β_2-agonists)
- Insulin
- Alkalemia

Extrarenal losses
- Skin – excessive sweating
- Gastrointestinal – diarrhea, fistulas

Renal losses
- Renal tubular acidosis
- Vomiting and nasogastric drainage
- Diuretics
- Bartter's syndrome
- Magnesium deficiency

Diagnosis. The differential diagnosis of the causes of hypokalemia is shown in Figure 2.2. Hypokalemia due to excessive loss is the most common cause; renal losses usually occur with the use of diuretics, metabolic acidosis and alkalosis. The most common transcellular shift occurs because of an abrupt increase in plasma catecholamines during an episode of intense stress, which activates the β_2-adrenergic receptor.

Treatment of hypokalemia depends on its severity and duration, and the underlying clinical context. Giving no treatment carries the risk of tachyarrhythmias, while aggressive treatment with potassium may result in hyperkalemia. Treatment is recommended for patients with a plasma potassium below 3 mmol/L regardless of the duration and the clinical context. In normal individuals, mild hypokalemia (plasma potassium 3.0–3.5 mmol/L), particularly if chronic, may not need treatment. On the other hand, even mild hypokalemia should be treated in patients receiving digoxin, individuals with structural or ischemic heart disease and patients with decompensated liver disease.

Oral therapy is preferable in chronic and/or mild hypokalemia. Intravenous potassium should be used cautiously (at a rate of

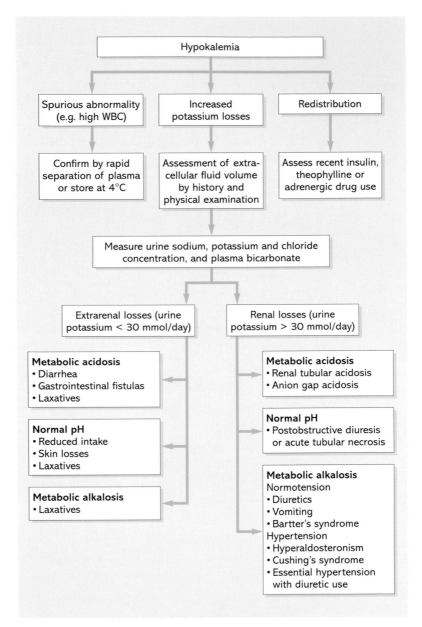

Figure 2.2 Diagnosis of cause of hypokalemia.

< 10 mmol/hour), under cardiac monitoring, and with follow-up
measurements of plasma potassium.

Hyperkalemia (plasma potassium > 5.0 mmol/L) is common (Table 2.6). Spurious hyperkalemia is not uncommon, and is usually the result of hemolysis caused by excessively tight or prolonged application of a tourniquet, underlying red-cell abnormalities or a extremely high platelet count.

The most common renal cause of hyperkalemia is chronic kidney disease (CKD), but this hyperkalemia usually only occurs when the GFR has fallen to less than 10 mL/minute. Aldosterone deficiency may be superimposed on CKD and is often acquired, for example with the use of drugs such as angiotensin-converting-enzyme (ACE) inhibitors and non-steroidal anti-inflammatory drugs (NSAIDs).

Clinical features. The clinical effects of hyperkalemia particularly affect the heart. ECG features include peaking or tenting of T waves, flattening of the P wave, prolongation of the PR interval and widening of the QRS complex (Figure 2.3). Ventricular fibrillation is the most severe consequence. Hyponatremic and hypocalcemic patients appear most vulnerable. Other manifestations include tingling,

TABLE 2.6

Causes of hyperkalemia

Increased intake	Reduced renal losses
• Potassium supplements	• Acute renal failure
• Medications (penicillin)	• Chronic renal failure
• Endogenous sources	• Medications
– rhabdomyolyis	– spironolactone, amiloride
– severe exercise	– angiotensin-converting-enzyme inhibitors or angiotensin-receptor blockers
– intravascular hemolysis	
Transcellular shifts	– ciclosporin A
• Non-selective β-blockers	– triamterene
• Hyperglycemia	
• Digoxin intoxication	
• Acidosis	

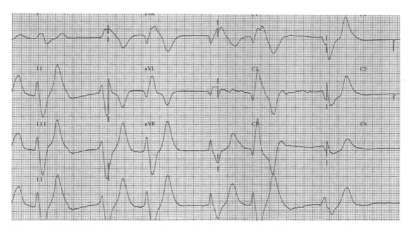

Figure 2.3 ECG in hyperkalemia showing large peaked T waves becoming sinusoidal.

paresthesias, weakness and flaccid paralysis, nausea, vomiting and abdominal pain.

Diagnosis. The key differential diagnosis is spurious hyperkalemia from hemolysis, often occurring during the phlebotomy.

Treatment of hyperkalemia depends on its severity and duration, and the clinical context. The presence of ECG changes and/or an absolute plasma potassium level above 7 mmol/L is an emergency. Immediate treatment with intravenous calcium chloride or calcium gluconate as a cardioprotective agent should be given, followed by steps to reduce the plasma potassium level either by inducing a transcellular shift of potassium from the extracellular to intracellular compartment (insulin/dextrose, salbutamol and treatment of acidosis if present) or by increasing potassium excretion (loop diuretics, sodium polystyrene or calcium resonium, or dialysis).

Disorders of calcium metabolism
The kidneys, intestine, bone and several hormones are involved in maintaining calcium balance.

Hypocalcemia. Since 70% of serum calcium is bound to albumin, the most common cause of hypocalcemia is a low plasma albumin concentration. This is false or spurious hypocalcemia (Table 2.7).

TABLE 2.7

Causes of hypocalcemia

- Primary hypoparathyroidism
  - idiopathic
  - postsurgical
- Pseudohypoparathyroidism
- Acute pancreatitis
- Hypocalcemia associated with malignancy

- Toxic shock syndrome
- Vitamin D deficiency
  - malabsorption
  - diet
  - chronic kidney disease
  - chronic hepatic disease
  - antiseizure therapy

Clinical features. The most common clinical manifestations of hypocalcemia are neuromuscular (e.g. tetany, seizures), ECG abnormalities (e.g. prolongation of the QTc and ST intervals, T wave peaking, T wave inversion) and psychiatric (e.g. confusion, depression, irritability). The classical clinical signs are Chvostek's and Trousseau's signs. Chvostek's sign is elicited by tapping the facial nerve immediately as it exits the auditory canal; however, Chvostek's sign may be positive in 10% of normal individuals. Trousseau's sign involves pumping a blood pressure cuff 3 mmHg above the systolic blood pressure and maintaining it for 10 minutes. A positive Trousseau's sign is present when the affected muscles undergo spasmodic contraction.

Diagnosis always requires measurement of calcium corrected for serum albumin.

Treatment. In general, patients with a calcium level corrected to below 1.75 mmol/L (7 mg/dL) or those with tetany, seizures and/or ECG abnormalities should be treated. Patients who are asymptomatic with a chronically low calcium level can be treated with oral calcium salts, vitamin D and the use of a thiazide to reduce renal excretion of calcium; calcium carbonate contains more elemental calcium than other salts. Patients with symptomatic and severe hypocalcemia must be given intravenous calcium with a bolus of calcium gluconate (10 mL of 10% calcium gluconate), under cardiac monitoring. Calcium gluconate is preferable to calcium chloride, because calcium chloride can cause tissue necrosis if accidentally extravasated.

Hypercalcemia. The most common cause of hypercalcemia among hospitalized patients is an underlying malignancy, whereas in a community outpatient setting the most common cause is primary hyperparathyroidism (Table 2.8).

Clinical features. Neurological features are usually the earliest manifestations of hypercalcemia, and gastrointestinal symptoms are often disabling (Table 2.9).

Diagnosis. All patients require a careful search for underlying malignancy and measurement of parathyroid hormone (PTH) level. In primary hyperparathyroidism the PTH is not suppressed by the raised calcium. Almost all other causes of hypercalcemia have a low or undetectable PTH level.

Treatment. Symptomatic patients with a serum calcium of 3.25 mmol/L (13 mg/dL) or more require urgent treatment, initially hydration with normal saline and diuretic therapy with furosemide. For patients with hypercalcemia secondary to a neoplasm, additional mithramycin, corticosteroids or bisphosphonates should be considered (cautiously in renal failure). Because bisphosphonates take 2–3 days to achieve maximum effect, calcitonin can be considered as a short-term therapy (effective within about 12 hours). Corticosteroids are commonly used for hematologic malignancies and are usually very effective.

TABLE 2.8

Causes of hypercalcemia

- Primary hyperparathyroidism
- Hypercalcemia of malignancy
- Thyrotoxicosis
- Sarcoidosis
- Tuberculosis
- Vitamin D intoxication
- Milk-alkali syndrome
- Immobilization
- Paget's disease
- Chronic renal failure (when treated for renal bone disease or with tertiary hyperparathyroidism)

TABLE 2.9

Clinical manifestations of hypercalcemia

Neurological	Gastrointestinal
• Headache	• Nausea
• Muscle weakness	• Vomiting
• Hypotonia	• Constipation
• Stupor	• Pancreatitis
• Confusion	**Cardiovascular**
• Coma	• Electrocardiographic changes
Psychiatric	**Renal**
• Depression	• Polyuria
• Irritability	• Reduced glomerular filtration rate
• Hallucinations	

Acid–base disorders

The normal range of the arterial pH is 7.36–7.44. Homeostatic mechanisms include systemic buffering of acid by both the circulation and bone, and the involvement of the respiratory and renal systems. Circulating and intracellular buffers quickly neutralize an acid load; however, the capacity of these buffering systems is soon exhausted in the absence of mechanisms to excrete acid. The two major organs that eliminate acid are the lungs and the kidneys. Acid is eliminated by the lungs in the form of carbon dioxide. The kidneys contribute by excreting acid as well as reclaiming bicarbonate.

Assessment of acid–base status. The first step in the evaluation of an acid–base problem is to measure serum electrolytes and arterial blood gases. After determining whether the patient has a metabolic/respiratory acidosis/alkalosis, the appropriateness of the secondary (or compensatory) physiological response should be assessed. In metabolic acidosis, calculation of the anion gap (i.e. serum sodium plus potassium minus serum chloride and bicarbonate) is very useful.

Metabolic acidosis is characterized by a primary decrease in the serum bicarbonate concentration. This occurs because of depletion or consumption of bicarbonate to buffer exogenous or endogenous generation of acid. Metabolic acidosis can be subdivided into that with an elevated anion gap and that with a normal anion gap (Table 2.10).

In proximal renal tubular acidosis, the primary defect is impaired reabsorption of bicarbonate by the proximal tubule. It is often associated with defective phosphate, glucose, urate and amino acid reabsorption. In distal renal tubular acidosis, the primary defect is an

TABLE 2.10

Causes of metabolic acidosis

Normal anion gap*

- Gastrointestinal
  - diarrhea
  - ureteroileostomy
- Renal
  - renal tubular acidosis
  - aldosterone deficiency (hyporeninemic hypoaldosteronism)
- Drugs
  - ammonium chloride
  - lysine or arginine hydrochloride

Elevated anion gap*

- Diabetic ketoacidosis
- Alcoholic ketoacidosis
- Starvation ketoacidosis
- Lactic acidosis
- Ingestion of toxins (methanol, ethylene glycol, salicylates, paraldehyde)
- Renal failure

*Anion gap = serum $(Na^+ + K^+) - (Cl^- + HCO_3^-)$

inability to acidify the urine maximally. Type 4 renal tubular acidosis is characterized by impaired urinary acidification caused by hypoaldosteronism. Lactic acidosis is often observed in critically ill hospitalized patients and reflects decreased tissue oxygenation.

The treatment of metabolic acidosis depends on the underlying cause and the severity of manifestations. In general, a pH of below 7.1, especially if it is associated with hemodynamic instability, should be treated by parenteral administration of sodium bicarbonate. In patients with chronic metabolic acidosis, such as a patient with a renal tubular acidosis, oral repletion with sodium bicarbonate is sufficient.

Metabolic alkalosis is characterized by a primary increase in the serum bicarbonate concentration. The most common causes are vomiting, diuretics and potassium depletion. The clinical features include muscle spasms, confusion, Chvostek's or Trousseau's signs, lethargy, seizures, coma and ventilatory depression.

After confirming the presence of metabolic alkalosis, the underlying cause should be identified together with the factors responsible for maintaining the alkalosis, especially extracellular volume depletion. The treatment of a metabolic alkalosis depends on identifying and remedying the underlying cause.

Respiratory acidosis and alkalosis occur as a consequence of primary abnormalities in the pulmonary mechanisms that maintain arterial pH. Respiratory acidosis results from impairment in the rate of alveolar ventilation. Acute respiratory acidosis is observed in situations in which there is a sudden depression of the medullary respiratory center, with paralysis of the muscles required for ventilation, or in airway obstruction. Chronic respiratory acidosis is observed in individuals with chronic airway disease.

Respiratory alkalosis occurs when hyperventilation reduces the arterial partial pressure of carbon dioxide and increases arterial pH. Acute respiratory alkalosis occurs most commonly as a result of the hyperventilation syndrome. It is characterized by lightheadedness, circumoral numbness and paresthesias; tetany may also occur.

Key points – electrolyte disturbance and acid–base disorders

- Electrolyte disturbances are very common and often iatrogenic.
- All electrolye disturbances require an accurate assessment of fluid balance.
- Intake and excretion of solutes, and drugs, must be considered when trying to identify causes.
- Correction should generally be cautious.

The term acute renal failure (ARF) describes a sudden reduction in GFR, occurring within days or weeks, that results in the accumulation of fluid and nitrogenous waste products usually excreted by the kidneys.

ARF is seen in up to 5% of hospital patients, and is far more common in the elderly. The incidence of severe ARF (serum creatinine > 5.7 mg/dL [500 µmol/L]) is about 140/million/year. ARF may result from poor perfusion of the kidneys (prerenal), intrinsic renal disease or urinary tract obstruction (postrenal). In general, prerenal ARF will recover rapidly once renal perfusion is reestablished. However, reversible prerenal ARF overlaps with, and may lead to, established ARF owing to ATN. In ATN, the degree of tubular damage is such that renal recovery is often delayed for 2 weeks or longer. ATN is by far the most common cause of ARF, and is often seen in postoperative patients in a hospital setting, and in those with severe infections or multisystem disease (Table 3.1).

Important questions

Is it truly prerenal ARF? It is important to establish whether patients with poor renal perfusion and accumulation of toxic metabolites have true prerenal ARF or whether they have established ATN. Urinary biochemistry may be helpful, since most patients with immediately reversible prerenal failure have a low urinary sodium concentration (< 20 mmol/L) and a high urine:plasma osmolality ratio (> 1.5). In practice, the management of patients will always include measures to increase renal perfusion, so the key issue is whether or not renal function shows a rapid response.

Were the kidneys previously normal? It is important to establish whether acute uremia is due to ARF in previously normal kidneys, or whether it represents a rapid decline against a background of CKD

TABLE 3.1

Causes of acute renal failure (ARF)

Prerenal

- Volume depletion (e.g. severe vomiting or diarrhea, burns, inappropriate diuretics)
- Hypotension (e.g. trauma, gastrointestinal hemorrhage)
- Cardiovascular (e.g. severe cardiac failure, arrhythmias)
- Drugs affecting renal perfusion (e.g. non-steroidal anti-inflammatory drugs, contrast media, ciclosporin, angiotensin-converting-enzyme inhibitors)
- Hepatorenal syndrome

Intrinsic ARF

- Acute tubular necrosis following prolonged ischemia
- Nephrotoxins (e.g. aminoglycosides, myoglobin, cisplatin, heavy metals, light chains in myeloma kidney)
- Acute interstitial nephritis due to drugs, infection or autoimmune diseases
- Glomerular damage (e.g. crescentic glomerulonephritis, vasculitis, hemolytic uremic syndrome)
- Vascular damage (e.g. renal artery occlusion, renal vein thrombosis, cholesterol emboli, scleroderma renal crisis, malignant hypertension)

Postrenal

- Ureteric obstruction (e.g. renal calculi, tumors, blood clots, retroperitoneal fibrosis)
- Bladder outlet obstruction (e.g. prostatic hypertrophy, bladder carcinoma)

(acute on chronic renal failure). The history and examination will provide clues, but renal ultrasonography will provide the most important information. In acute on chronic renal failure, renal abnormalities, such as small kidneys in chronic glomerulonephritis or large cystic kidneys in adult polycystic kidney disease, will almost always be present. It is necessary to decide whether the acute uremic episode represents the natural history of these diseases, or whether exacerbating factors that may be reversible are responsible.

Is an obstruction present? If obstruction could be the cause of ARF, kidney function may improve rapidly once the obstruction is relieved. This should be revealed by renal ultrasonography.

Is intrinsic renal disease requiring urgent therapy present? Tubulointerstitial nephritis or glomerulonephritis may be suggested by abnormal findings on urine microscopy (e.g. hematuria, proteinuria, red-cell casts).

Is acute vascular occlusion present? Possible occlusion should be assessed by Doppler ultrasonography of the renal artery and veins. If it is strongly suspected, more accurate imaging (for example using magnetic resonance angiography) should be performed.

Intrinsic renal disease

Established ARF is most often due to ATN. The most common cause of ATN is prolonged renal ischemia due to reduced renal perfusion, which may be a result of volume depletion, septicemia, cardiac failure or renal artery obstruction. Tubular damage is often caused by exogenous toxins, such as NSAIDs, heavy metals and contrast agents. Endogenous tubular toxins, such as myoglobin (in rhabdomyolysis), hemoglobin (in hemolysis) or immunoglobulin light chains (in myeloma), are also important causes. It is essential to look for hematuria, urinary casts and proteinuria, which suggest a diagnosis of glomerulonephritis or tubulointerstitial nephritis. In these circumstances, renal biopsy may be indicated. When the cause of ARF is unclear, a number of blood tests may be helpful (Table 3.2).

Postrenal acute renal failure

Postrenal ARF is usually the result of obstruction of the lower urinary tract by calculi, tumors or prostatic hypertrophy. In most cases (but not all), lower tract obstruction will lead to dilatation of the renal pelvis, which is visible on ultrasonography. ARF due to obstruction generally

TABLE 3.2

Blood tests in acute renal failure

Test	Diagnosis
Creatine kinase	Rhabdomyolysis
Eosinophilia	Acute interstitial nephritis Cholesterol emboli
Anti-DNA antibodies	SLE
Low complement levels	SLE Cryoglobulinemia Cholesterol emboli
Cryoglobulins	Cryoglobulinemia
Antineutrophil cytoplasm antibodies	Systemic vasculitis
Anti-GBM antibodies	Goodpasture's syndrome
Serum electrophoresis (paraprotein)	Multiple myeloma

GBM, glomerular basement membrane; SLE, systemic lupus erythematosus.

resolves once it is relieved by placement of a bladder catheter or percutaneous nephrostomy. Prolonged obstruction may lead to irreversible renal damage. Less commonly, intrarenal obstruction occurs as a result of deposition of crystals in the tubules (e.g. oxalate in ethylene glycol poisoning).

Management

Management of ARF includes the treatment of any underlying cause, general medical management of renal failure and, if necessary, renal replacement therapy (dialysis). In prerenal failure, correction of volume depletion, using central venous pressure monitoring when necessary, should result in rapid recovery of renal function (Table 3.3). However, once ATN has developed, and in other causes of ARF, the patient will often be oliguric for several days or weeks.

Patients with ATN lose the ability both to concentrate and dilute the urine, and will pass a constant volume with inappropriate osmolality. Accurate measurement of urine output is essential to prevent volume

TABLE 3.3

Management of acute renal failure

- Accurate control of fluid balance (avoid volume overload or depletion)
- Potassium restriction
- Daily measurement of serum electrolytes
- Nutritional support
- Careful drug dosing
- Avoidance of nephrotoxic drugs
- Specific treatment of underlying intrinsic renal disease where appropriate
- Dialysis or hemofiltration

overload or depletion. Most patients are oliguric and, in general, should be provided with a volume of fluid equal to the output on the previous day, plus at the very least an extra 500 mL if pyrexia is present. Since the situation may change rapidly, daily clinical assessment together with CVP monitoring and measurement of body weight is required. Although diuretics do not alter the course or outcome of ARF, high-dose diuretics may convert oliguric ARF to non-oliguric ARF, which is worthwhile if dialysis is not readily available. There is no evidence in favor of using low-dose dopamine infusions; indeed, there is good evidence of a lack of benefit.

Potassium restriction is nearly always necessary and is typically limited to less than 50 mmol/day. In the acute situation, hyperkalemia may be managed with dextrose/insulin infusions and administration of calcium gluconate. In the slightly longer term, potassium-binding resins can be used if dialysis is not immediately available. Sodium intake should be restricted to about 80 mmol/day, depending on losses. Serum potassium and sodium concentrations should be assessed daily. Acidosis may be limited by protein restriction, though a daily intake of at least approximately 1 g of high-quality protein per kilogram of body weight is necessary to maintain adequate nutrition. Sodium bicarbonate may be used to treat acidosis, but has the potential disadvantage that it may worsen sodium overload.

As many of the drugs prescribed for patients with ARF are excreted via the kidney, doses must be adjusted and drug levels monitored accordingly. Nephrotoxic drugs, such as NSAIDs and aminoglycosides, should be avoided. Patients in renal failure are susceptible to infection, so it is important to take great care of intravenous lines, to perform regular cultures of body fluids and to use antibiotics early. As gastrointestinal hemorrhage is another potential cause of morbidity in ARF, prophylactic treatment to reduce acid secretion is generally indicated. It is important to maintain adequate nutrition, preferably via the enteral route, but using parenteral nutrition if necessary.

Dialysis is indicated to treat the clinical consequences of uremia and to control electrolyte, acid–base and fluid balance. In oliguric or anuric patients, the fluid intake required for feeding generally means that dialysis will be necessary (Table 3.4). Peritoneal dialysis is usually only performed when hemodialysis is unavailable. In patients who are hemodynamically unstable, particularly those in intensive care, continuous dialysis techniques (e.g. hemodiafiltration) are better tolerated than intermittent hemodialysis and allow more effective control of fluid balance.

Specific treatments

Acute renal artery thrombosis (of a single functioning kidney) may be treated surgically, or by angioplasty and stenting. In rhabdomyolysis with myoglobulinuria, alkaline diuresis may prevent the development of

TABLE 3.4

Indications for dialysis in acute renal failure

- Presence of clinical features of uremia (e.g. pericarditis, encephalopathy)
- Fluid retention leading to pulmonary edema
- Severe hyperkalemia unresponsive to medical management
- Acidosis that cannot be controlled by sodium bicarbonate
- Biochemical results indicating severe renal failure (urea > 30 mmol/L [84 mg/dL], creatinine > 500 μmol/L [5.7 mg/dL])

severe renal failure, but must be undertaken with care in oliguric patients. Acute tubulointerstitial nephritis may respond to a short course of high-dose corticosteroids, though no controlled trials have been undertaken to support this approach. ARF due to crescentic glomerulonephritis may respond to treatment with prednisolone and cyclophosphamide, together with the addition of plasma exchange (see Chapter 6). Hemolytic uremic syndrome (HUS) may respond to plasma exchange with fresh frozen plasma.

Outcome

Most patients with ATN should recover renal function, provided that they survive the underlying illness. Similarly, most patients will recover from acute interstitial nephritis. Recovery from glomerulonephritis is more variable; patients usually recover if treated early, but are likely to remain dependent on dialysis if treated late or inadequately.

Survival in ARF depends on the cause, and mortality remains high (40–80%) in patients with multiple organ failure. Death is likely if ARF is associated with failure of more than three other organ systems. In patients acquiring ARF in the community, however, mortality is much lower (10–30%).

Key points – acute renal failure

- Acute renal failure (ARF) is common and often reversible if diagnosed promptly.
- Recognition of volume depletion or overload is crucial in the early management of ARF.
- Drug doses often need to be modified.
- Acute tubular necrosis has no specific treatment other than volume control, and there is no benefit in the routine use of dopamine or furosemide.

Key references

Esson ML, Schrier RW. Diagnosis
and treatment of acute tubular
necrosis. *Ann Intern Med*
2002;137:744–52.

Schrier RW, Wang W, Poole B, Mitra
A. Acute renal failure: definitions,
diagnosis, pathogenesis, and therapy.
J Clin Invest 2004;114:5–14; *J Clin
Invest* 2004;114:598.

Chronic kidney disease

Chronic kidney disease (CKD) is common and underrecognized. It can be defined as kidney damage present for at least 3 months, with either structural or functional abnormalities of the kidney with or without decreased GFR. In the early stages of CKD, evidence of kidney damage (e.g. proteinuria, cysts, biopsy changes) may be seen in the presence of a normal GFR (> 60 mL/minute/1.73 m^2), while the later stages are characterized by greater functional impairment with the GFR falling to below 60 mL/minute/1.73 m^2 (Table 4.1).

Epidemiology

Approximately 20 million people in the USA are in CKD stages 1–4, which far exceeds the 300 000 patients receiving hemodialysis. In the UK the numbers are smaller (about 20 000 patients on dialysis) but the

TABLE 4.1

Definition and stages of chronic kidney disease*

GFR (mL/minute/1.73 m^2)	Disease stage	Comments
> 90	1	It no kidney damage by any criterion is present, this is normal
60–89	2	If no kidney damage is present, this represents decreased GFR only, which might be normal for age
30–59	3	Always abnormal
15–29	4	Always abnormal
< 15 or dialysis	5	End-stage renal failure

*Modified from the National Kidney Foundation (USA) Kidney Disease Outcomes Quality Initiative (K/DOQI) guidelines, 2002.
GFR, glomerular filtration rate.

huge excess of patients with CKD is similar (estimated at over 2 million). This is particularly important, because much of the damage caused by CKD occurs early, when interventions may slow progressive renal damage, prevent left ventricular hypertrophy, minimize vascular disease and improve quality of life.

The incidence of CKD leading to dialysis varies worldwide; the number of patients per million population starting dialysis each year is 300 in the USA compared with 230 in Japan and 110 in the UK. The prevalence of end-stage renal failure (ESRF) also varies; in the USA, 1 in 1000 of the population are receiving treatment for ESRF (dialysis or transplantation) and, overall, the number of patients per million population is 1131 compared with 1397 in Japan, 690 in Canada, 634 in France, 530 in Australia and 498 in the UK and 223 in Poland. Reasons for this wide variation include both patient factors (e.g. the prevalence of diabetes) and external factors (e.g. the availability of dialysis and the number of nephrologists).

The three most important causes of CKD are diabetes, glomerulonephritis and hypertension (and other vascular disease), but the primary cause does vary geographically (Table 4.2). However, renal failure resulting from diabetes and hypertension is potentially preventable (see Chapter 5), and many causes of glomerulonephritis can be treated if diagnosed at an early stage (see Chapter 6).

Clinical features

CKD usually presents with non-specific symptoms caused by renal failure and the underlying disease, or is discovered by chance following a routine blood or urine test. Specific symptoms usually develop only in severe renal failure. The most common symptoms in late renal failure include anorexia, nausea, vomiting, fatigue, weakness, pruritus, edema, lethargy, dyspnea, insomnia, muscle cramps, pulmonary edema, nocturia, polyuria and headache. Sexual dysfunction is rarely reported voluntarily, but is common. Hiccups, pericarditis, coma and seizures are seldom seen except in developing countries when renal disease presents very late.

Signs of CKD include skin pigmentation or excoriation, anemia, hypertension, postural hypotension, edema, left ventricular

TABLE 4.2

Causes of end-stage renal failure (data from renal registries)

Primary cause	Australia and New Zealand	Europe	USA
Arteriopathic renal disease and hypertension	14%	13%	30%
Glomerulonephritis	35%	12%	14%
Diabetes	20%	18%	36%
Infective or obstructive nephropathies	10%	13%	4%
Congenital disease	0.5%	0.7%	0.2%
Familial or hereditary disease	9%	9%	3%
Neoplasms	1%	3%	2%
Miscellaneous	3%	2%	2%
Unknown	7%	29%	9%

hypertrophy, peripheral vascular disease, lung crackles, pleural effusions, peripheral neuropathy and urine abnormalities (presence of blood or protein).

Diagnosis

Recognition of abnormal renal function is the key to the diagnosis of CKD. However, blood urea nitrogen (BUN or serum urea) is an extremely poor marker of renal function, because it varies significantly with hydration status and diet, it is not produced constantly and it is reabsorbed by the kidney. Historically, serum creatinine has been used, but this also has significant limitations, particularly the fact that the level can remain within the normal range despite the loss of over 50% of renal function. A 'gold-standard' measurement is an isotopic GFR, but this is expensive and not available in community settings. It is now clear that calculated GFR using a formula based on serum creatinine is a reasonable compromise, and can be a valid, reliable, repeatable and reasonably accurate measure of true GFR in patients with renal impairment (see Chapter 2). Measurement of serum cystatin C is also a reliable marker of GFR, but this test is not yet widely available.

Management

CKD is generally a progressive disease (Figure 4.1), though the rate of decline in renal function varies between patients. In the last decade, it has become clear that, regardless of the underlying cause of the renal disease, the factors that will determine the likelihood of progression to ESRF are:

- the level of proteinuria
- the initial degree of renal impairment
- blood pressure.

Treatments aimed at reducing proteinuria and vigorously controlling blood pressure have been shown to slow or even halt the decline in renal function and to reduce the vascular complications, which are the leading cause of death in CKD. Even a relatively small change in the progression of renal failure has enormous implications both for the individual patient (quality of life declines significantly once dialysis is needed), and for governments or insurers (dialysis is expensive and even a small delay before it is necessary saves millions of dollars a year).

The management of CKD is summarized in Tables 4.3 and 4.4. Blood pressure targets are extremely low and some drugs are

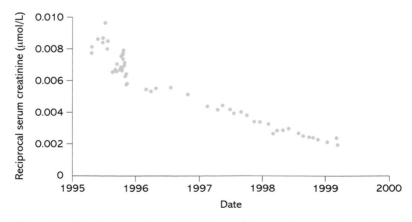

Figure 4.1 Steady decline in renal function over time as shown by the reciprocal serum creatinine plot.

TABLE 4.3

Clinical approach in chronic kidney disease*

	GFR (mL/minute/ 1.73 m²)	Management
Stage 1		
Kidney damage with normal GFR	≥ 90	Diagnose and treat underlying cause, treat comorbid conditions, slow progression by controlling blood pressure and reducing proteinuria, reduce cardiovascular risk
Stage 2		
Kidney damage with mild decrease in GFR	60–89	As for stage 1 and estimate progression
Stage 3		
Moderate decrease in GFR	30–59	Prevent and treat complications
Stage 4		
Severe reduction in GFR	15–29	Prepare for renal replacement therapy (dialysis or transplantation)
Stage 5		
Kidney failure	< 15 (or dialysis)	Renal replacement therapy

*Modified from the National Kidney Foundation (USA) Kidney Disease Outcomes Quality Initiative (K/DOQI) guidelines, 2002.

undoubtedly more beneficial than others (e.g. angiotensin-converting-enzyme [ACE] inhibitors in patients with proteinuria), though in reality all classes of drug need to be used for blood-pressure control, and most patients will require at least three or four drugs. Evidence suggests that there is no lower limit to the blood pressure which will slow progression of renal disease, and current targets lie between

TABLE 4.4

Management of chronic kidney disease

Blood pressure

- Aim for < 130/80 mmHg
- Angiotensin-converting-enzyme (ACE) inhibitors slow renal progression independently of their blood-pressure-lowering effect and should be used in all patients if tolerated and if renal artery stenosis not present

Proteinuria

- Reduce proteinuria as much as possible; ACE inhibitors and angiotensin-receptor antagonists are particularly effective, but diltiazem, verapamil and thiazide diuretics can also be used

Conventional cardiovascular risk factors

- Stop smoking
- Eat a low-salt diet
- Take regular exercise
- Hypercholesterolemia, if present (though rare in chronic kidney disease, and most trials excluded patients with renal failure), should be treated with a statin
- Antioxidants (vitamin E) may prevent cardiovascular disease
- No evidence of benefit of folic acid in hyperhomocysteinemia

Anemia

- Early erythropoietin therapy may prevent left ventricular hypertrophy, but precise timing of initiation uncertain

Acidosis

- May hasten renal progression, contribute to bone disease and muscle breakdown
- Treat with sodium bicarbonate, but can cause fluid overload and worsen hypertension

Hyperphosphatemia

- Occurs late in chronic kidney disease (usually stage 4 or 5)
- Treat with dietary restriction and phosphate binders

Malnutrition

- Must be avoided, although protein restriction can slow progression

125/75 mmHg and 130/80 mmHg. Patients with diabetes undoubtedly benefit from renin-angiotensin blockade with either an ACE inhibitor, an angiotensin-receptor blocker (ARB) or a combination of both. For patients on dialysis, the most important factor in controlling blood pressure is to control salt (and water) intake and body fluid volume. A full discussion of hypertension and kidney disease will be found in Chapter 5.

Evidence shows that early referral to a nephrologist reduces morbidity and early mortality in ESRF. Plans for renal replacement therapy when it becomes necessary require careful consideration. Patients being considered for predialysis transplantation, from either a living donor or a cadaver, require a full assessment of their suitability for the procedure. Patients need to be educated about the methods of dialysis (and conservative care), preservation of forearm veins and, if opting for hemodialysis, early formation of an arteriovenous fistula to avoid the need for intravenous dialysis catheters. Patients should also be vaccinated against hepatitis B early in CKD, when the immune response is better preserved.

Complications

CKD leads to a variety of complications, which can all cause considerable morbidity (Table 4.5). One of the major aims of care in patients with CKD is to minimize these complications, even if the underlying renal disease cannot be treated. Many complications are common to both CKD and patients established on dialysis. Further investigations to identify complications of renal disease and to establish the underlying cause are summarized in Table 4.6.

Anemia is universal in ESRF and is largely due to a relative lack of erythropoietin. It usually develops when the GFR falls below 35 mL/minute and worsens as the GFR declines further. It is not solely due to erythropoietin deficiency; red-cell survival is shortened in uremia, iron deficiency is common, and vitamin B_{12} and folate deficiencies also occur. Furthermore, patients may have a hemoglobinopathy or hemolysis, and hyperparathyroidism inhibits red-cell production. There is a strong association between anemia and

TABLE 4.5

Complications of chronic kidney disease

Complication	Effect
Anemia	Left ventricular hypertrophy, fatigue, impaired cognitive functioning
Hypertension	Left ventricular hypertrophy, heart failure, stroke, cardiovascular disease
Calcium phosphate loading	Cardiovascular and cerebrovascular disease, arthropathy, soft tissue calcification
Renal bone disease	Bone pain, fractures
Dialysis amyloid	Bone pain, arthropathy, carpal tunnel syndrome
Fluid overload	Pulmonary edema, hypertension
Malnutrition	Increased morbidity and mortality, infections, poor wound healing

risk of death in ESRF, and an association with increasing cardiovascular morbidity and mortality in CKD. Correcting anemia leads to major improvements in quality of life, exercise capacity, cognitive function, nutrition, sexual function, sleep, left ventricular hypertrophy and cardiac output in ESRF, and the benefits most likely extend to CKD as well.

Investigations to exclude other causes of anemia in CKD patients should include blood film, red-cell indices, white cells and platelets, serum iron, ferritin and transferrin saturation, serum vitamin B_{12} and red-cell folate. If no cause is found, erythropoietin deficiency is likely and replacement therapy can be considered. Several erythropoietic agents (e.g. Eprex, Epogen, Procrit, NeoRecormon, Aranesp) are now licensed and widely available, all of which are effective (but expensive). They are usually given 1–3 times/week by subcutaneous or intravenous injection. (Eprex is only given intravenously as it has been associated with immunological toxicity.) Patients need replete iron stores in order to benefit from erythropoietin and therefore should usually be given

iron intravenously.

TABLE 4.6

Investigation of complications in chronic kidney disease

Investigation	Comment
Serum sodium	Usually normal, but may be low
Serum potassium	Raised, often with a precipitant, but usually controllable by diet
Serum bicarbonate	Low, may need treatment
Serum albumin	Low levels at start of dialysis strongly associated with poor prognosis. Reflects both inflammation and malnutrition
Serum calcium	May be normal, low or high
Serum phosphate	Usually high and leads to vascular calcification
Serum alkaline phosphatase	Raised when bone disease develops
Plasma glucose	To detect undiagnosed diabetes or assess diabetic control
Serum parathyroid hormone	Rises progressively with declining renal function
Serum cholesterol and triglycerides	Dyslipidemia common, often with raised triglycerides
Hemoglobin	Low and falls with progressive renal failure
Serum ferritin	Large iron stores needed to utilize prescribed erythropoietin
White cells and platelets	Usually normal
Clotting	Normal
HLA tissue typing	Performed as a prelude to transplantation
Hepatitis serology	Ensure not infected and vaccinate against hepatitis B
HIV serology	Performed before dialysis or transplantation
ECG and echocardiography	To detect left ventricular hypertrophy and ischemia, and to assess cardiac function

CONTINUED

TABLE 4.6 (CONTINUED)

Investigation of complications in chronic kidney disease

| Renal ultrasound | To confirm diagnosis or exclude treatable acute renal failure |

ECG, electrocardiogram; HIV, human immunodeficiency virus; HLA, human leukocyte antigen.

Cardiovascular complications. Cardiovascular disease is the most common cause of death in patients with CKD, and cardiovascular mortality is doubled in patients with a GFR below 70 mL/minute (i.e. quite moderate renal impairment).

The risk factors for cardiovascular disease in CKD are summarized in Table 4.7; the risks increase as renal function deteriorates. The major cardiovascular outcomes include stroke, sudden death, arrhythmia, myocardial infarction, ischemic heart disease, cardiac arrest, hypertension, pericarditis, left ventricular hypertrophy and vascular calcification (Figure 4.2).

No randomized controlled trials of interventions specifically in patients with renal failure have been carried out, but it is possible to suggest some guidelines for reducing the risk of cardiovascular complications (Table 4.8).

In general, the management of cardiovascular disease is similar in patients with and without renal disease. Care needs to be taken over drug dosing (e.g. avoiding long-acting β-blockers). Patients with CKD undergoing angiography should be protected from contrast nephropathy by hydration and possibly the use of N-acetylcysteine. Anemia should be corrected with erythropoietin. Although thrombolysis and surgery can be safely carried out, surgery can cause hypotension, leading to acute deterioration in renal function. Control of calcium and phosphate balance is critical in later renal failure to avoid vascular calcification and stiffening.

Hypertension can be both a cause and consequence of renal disease, and uncontrolled hypertension is the most important factor contributing to the rate of progression of renal damage, whatever the

TABLE 4.7

Risk factors for cardiovascular disease in chronic kidney disease

General risk factors	Risk factors unique to renal failure
• Age	• Anemia
• Male sex	• Hyperparathyroidism
• Smoking	• Uremia
• Family history	• Hyperphosphatemia
• Thrombogenic factors	• Malnutrition
• Obesity	• Arteriovenous fistulas
	• Volume overload

Risk factors with increased prevalence in renal failure

- Hypertension
- Diabetes
- Physical inactivity
- Left ventricular hypertrophy
- Cholesterol
- Lipoprotein (a)
- Homocysteine

original cause (see Chapter 5). In addition to slowing or preventing the progression of chronic kidney disease, tight blood pressure control also reduces overall cardiovascular outcomes and improves left ventricular hypertrophy.

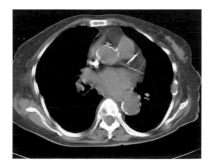

Figure 4.2 Computerized tomography scan showing coronary artery and aortic calcification in a patient with end-stage renal failure.

TABLE 4.8

Measures to reduce cardiovascular outcomes in chronic kidney disease

Risk factor	Target and/or treatment
Smoking	Smoking cessation
Hypertension	Reduce blood pressure to < 140/85 mmHg
Diabetes	Reduce glycosylated hemoglobin to < 7.5%
Thrombogenic factors	Aspirin, 75 mg/day, unless contraindicated
Obesity	Appropriate dietary advice
Physical inactivity	Encourage exercise
Left ventricular hypertrophy	Control blood pressure, treat anemia
Cholesterol	Reduce to < 5.0 mmol/L (statins in all cases?)
Lipoprotein (a)	No treatment available
Anemia	Increase Hb to > 11 g/dL with iron and EPO
Hyperparathyroidism	Reduce PTH to < 200 pg/mL with vitamin D analogs or calcimimetics
Hyperphosphatemia	Reduce PO_4 to < 2.0 mmol/L with PO_4 binders
Uremia	Ensure dialysis adequate
Malnutrition	Improve nutrition as much as possible

Renal bone disease. A number of factors contribute to renal bone disease (Table 4.9). Furthermore, the complications of calcium and phosphate balance not only affect the skeleton, but are now known to contribute to vascular disease. Osteodystrophy develops at a relatively early stage of renal failure, when the GFR falls below 30–40 mL/minute, and all patients with ESRF develop some manifestations of bone disease. The main underlying cause is decreased production of 1,25-dihydroxyvitamin D, which causes hypocalcemia and leads to increased secretion of PTH (Figure 4.3). Phosphate retention also begins relatively early and further stimulates PTH

TABLE 4.9

Factors contributing to bone renal disease

- Hyperparathyroidism
- Acidosis
- Low levels of vitamin D (in some patients)
- Suppressed parathyroid activity (after treatment)
- Aluminum accumulation (now rare)
- Osteoporosis in elderly patients
- Osteopenia caused by corticosteroids used to treat initial disease or for transplantation

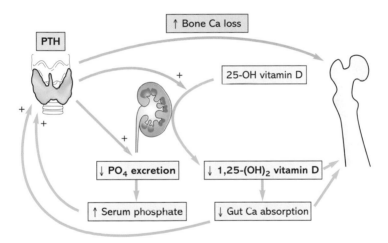

Figure 4.3 In renal bone disease, decreased production of 1,25-dihydroxy-vitamin D stimulates parathyroid hormone (PTH) secretion, and causes hypocalcemia, further increasing secretion of PTH. Phosphate retention also stimulates PTH secretion. Bone disease is a consequence of both high PTH and low vitamin D levels.

secretion. Hyperparathyroidism initially corrects the biochemical abnormalities by increasing phosphate excretion, stimulating vitamin D synthesis and increasing serum calcium levels, but at the expense of the skeleton, which can develop osteitis fibrosa. Independently, vitamin D deficiency can lead to osteomalacia.

Symptoms of renal bone disease include pruritus and bone and joint pain. Among the biochemical features are raised serum phosphate, raised serum PTH, and a low or low-normal serum calcium. Calcium levels rise only after treatment with vitamin D analogs or calcium salts. Elevated levels of alkaline phosphatase are seen in established osteomalacia.

The aims of treatment include prevention of hyperphosphatemia, maintenance of normal serum calcium and inhibition of hyperparathyroidism. Patients need comprehensive advice about low-phosphate diets, and usually need to take phosphate binders with meals to reduce absorption of dietary phosphate. (Historically, aluminum salts were given, until it was recognized that aluminum itself caused neurological damage, anemia and bone disease.) Calcium salts have also been widely used, because they also treat hypocalcemia. However, recent evidence suggests that the calcium absorbed in this way may contribute to vascular calcification and increased cardiovascular morbidity and mortality in ESRF. Non-calcium phosphate binders (sevelamer and lanthanum) are increasingly being used.

Vitamin D analogs can effectively suppress PTH, but often at the price of encouraging hypercalcemia. Newer calcimimetic agents (cinacalcet) can also lower PTH levels without affecting serum calcium. Some patients require parathyroidectomy if all else fails.

Dialysis amyloid is a complication that affects all patients who have been on dialysis for over 20 years. It is caused by the accumulation of β_2-microglobulin, which is deposited as amyloid in joints and bone. The initial manifestation is usually carpal tunnel syndrome, which often occurs about 7 years after the start of dialysis. Later, joint pains occur, which start in the shoulders and are worse at night, together with tenosynovitis of the finger flexors, destructive spondylarthropathy of the cervical spine and, occasionally, soft tissue accumulation. Radiographs may show bone cysts.

Dialysis amyloid can be treated only by renal transplantation, and symptoms and signs may take years to abate; other treatments are palliative. It must, therefore, be prevented by using newer dialysis membranes and techniques (diafiltration) for hemodialysis, and longer hours of dialysis.

Fluid overload, diet and nutrition. Patients with ESRF are often almost anuric and must therefore watch their fluid intake carefully. This is particularly a problem for patients on hemodialysis. Fluid overload can lead to pulmonary edema, peripheral edema and hypertension. Some patients with CKD retain salt and water, and develop fluid overload requiring diuretics, while others lose salt and water, and become volume depleted, possibly requiring treatment with oral sodium bicarbonate.

Malnutrition is a particularly important problem in ESRF, and affects 40–50% of patients (Table 4.10). It is associated with an increased number of infections, muscle wasting, poor wound healing, and increased morbidity and mortality. The complexities of maintaining nutritional requirements in ESRF while limiting protein, salt, phosphate and fluid intake require the assistance of dietitians from an early stage in CKD. Serum albumin is often used as an indication of nutritional state, but it must be remembered that it also falls in inflammatory conditions. A global evaluation of nutrition is much more useful, for example the subjective global assessment, which incorporates measures of dietary intake, comorbidity, functional capabilities and changes in body weight.

Sexual, psychological and social complications. Sexual dysfunction is extremely common in patients with CKD. Decreased libido, erectile dysfunction, amenorrhea and infertility may occur, often compounded by depression, anxiety and changes in body image.

Depression affects up to 60% of patients with ESRF and can manifest in many ways, many of which can also be consequences of uremia. Treatment involves high-quality dialysis and psychological or pharmacological interventions as appropriate. The side effects of psychotropic drugs are often increased in renal failure.

Many patients in ESRF also face changes in employment, social status, ability to obtain insurance and mortgages, and ability to travel. Social support is therefore immensely important and increases survival.

TABLE 4.10

Causes of malnutrition in end-stage renal failure

Factors increasing nutrient requirements

Metabolic abnormalities

- Altered amino acid and lipid metabolism
- Impaired glucose tolerance
- Hyperparathyroidism
- Metabolic acidosis
- Carnitine depletion
- Increased cytokine and leptin activity
- Uremia

Concomitant disease

- Cardiovascular disease
- Sepsis
- Inflammation

Factors decreasing food intake

Anorexia

- Nausea
- Fatigue
- Taste changes
- Anemia
- Medications

Gastrointestinal disturbances

- Phosphate binders
- Hypoalbuminemia
- Antibiotics
- Uremic and diabetic gastroparesis

Psychosocial and socioeconomic

- Depression
- Anxiety
- Ignorance
- Loneliness
- Alcohol or drug abuse
- Poverty

Key points – chronic kidney disease

- Chronic kidney disease is very common, especially the early stages.
- Early interventions can prevent progressive decline in renal function and complications.
- Blood pressure control is crucial, and very low targets should be set.
- Cardiovascular risk factors need aggressive management.
- Anemia and bone disease may require treatment before dialysis is necessary.

The epidemic of chronic kidney disease. The incidence of CKD is relatively very high in some populations such as Indo-Asians, African-Americans and Afro-Caribbeans, Native Americans and Australian Aboriginals. Much of this CKD is due to type 2 diabetes and to hypertension, but there are also unknown causes of renal failure. In developing countries an epidemic of CKD has begun, often associated with a westernization (i.e. degradation) of diet and an increase in population obesity and type 2 diabetes. Unless – ideally – the rise is halted, or else the disease is properly treated, we may expect a huge increase in the potential need for renal replacement therapies and in death in developing countries that cannot afford dialysis.

Key references

Levey AS, Bosch JP, Lewis JB et al.; Modification of Diet in Renal Disease Study Group. A more accurate method to estimate glomerular filtration rate from serum creatinine: a new prediction equation. *Ann Intern Med* 1999; 130:461–70.

UK Renal Registry
www.renalreg.com

www.kidney.org/professionals/kdoqi/index.cfm

5 | Hypertension and diabetic nephropathy

Hypertension

Hypertension is the most common chronic disease in the Western world; by the age of 60 years, over 50% of the population will have developed high blood pressure. Hypertension is even more common among patients with CKD; by the time patients develop ESRF, over 80% have elevated blood pressure, and hypertension accounts for approximately 20% of all cases of kidney failure. After diabetes mellitus, hypertension is the second leading cause of kidney failure in the USA, though it is less common as a formal cause of ESRF in Europe.

Hypertension is arbitrarily defined as a pressure of 140/90 mmHg or more (Table 5.1); a new category of risk termed prehypertension has been created in recent US guidelines. After the age of 60 years, most of the population either has hypertension or is at risk of developing it. However, only 59% of these individuals receive treatment, and of these, only 34% are well controlled. The situation is much worse for individuals with CKD; only 14% achieve a blood pressure level of 140/90 mmHg or lower.

TABLE 5.1

Classification of hypertension

Classification	Blood pressure Systolic (mmHg)	Diastolic (mmHg)
Normal	< 120	< 80
Prehypertension	120–139	80–89
Hypertension		
• stage I	140–159	90–99
• stage II	≥ 160	≥ 100

Adapted from the Joint National Committee on the Prevention, Detection, Evaluation and Treatment of High Blood Pressure. *Hypertension* 2003;42:1206–52.

Essential hypertension represents an elevation in systemic arterial blood pressure in the absence of a known etiology and accounts for 90% of cases, with most of the remainder being caused by renal disease. Endocrine or metabolic causes are rare.

Hypertension associated with parenchymal kidney disease represents a potent vicious cycle; it is both a consequence of CKD and a cause of progressive renal damage. Evidence from many studies shows that treatment of hypertension is crucial to slowing progression of kidney disease, particularly among those with significant proteinuria (> 1 g/24 hours).

The major complications associated with elevated blood pressure are an increased risk of cardiovascular and cerebrovascular disease, kidney failure (Figure 5.1), retinopathy and peripheral vascular disease.

Since hypertension is a common chronic condition, the evaluation and treatment of comorbidities associated with hypertension should be an integral part of management. In particular, recent evidence from the

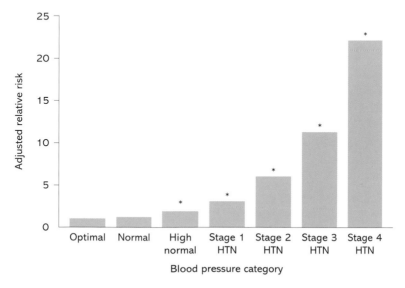

Figure 5.1 A rise in blood pressure is a strong independent risk factor for end-stage renal failure. *$p < 0.001$ versus optimal.

Data from Klag MJ, Whelton PK, Randall BL et al. Blood pressure and end-stage renal disease in men. *N Engl J Med* 1996;334:13–18.

Anglo-Scandinavian Cardiac Outcome Trial (ASCOT) attests to the importance of treating hypertensive patients with a statin. In this study, among hypertensive patients with normal or only moderately raised levels of cholesterol, patients receiving atorvastatin were 30% less likely to suffer coronary events and 27% less likely to have a stroke.

Diagnosis. The widespread availability of ambulatory electronic and manual devices, and the proliferation of automated devices, have made the standardization of blood pressure measurement critical to diagnosis and subsequent follow-up. Blood pressure should be measured using the correct size of cuff, with the patient at rest in the correct position, either seated or supine. Two measurements should be taken at least 2 minutes apart in order to reduce variability. In addition, blood pressure should be measured two or three times separated by an interval of several weeks before a definitive diagnosis is made, unless the initial measurement is sufficiently high (> 180/100 mmHg) to justify immediate treatment.

Investigations should be undertaken to identify the underlying cause, assess the extent of target organ damage, and recognize the presence of comorbid conditions that should influence the aggressiveness of therapy. Routine laboratory evaluation should include urinalysis, blood glucose, complete blood count, urea and electrolytes, lipid profile and an ECG. In most patients, urine protein measurement is a useful indicator of kidney involvement. Screening for microalbuminuria is recommended in type 2 diabetics at the time of diagnosis and in type 1 diabetics at 5 years after the initial diagnosis.

Management. Antihypertensive therapy is beneficial in reducing both cardiovascular and renal events, as well as lowering mortality. In patients with CKD, treating hypertension is important in slowing disease progression and in reducing cardiovascular risk. In patients with ESRF, the focus should be directed towards reducing cardiovascular morbidity. Patients with CKD require aggressive management of blood pressure, with a target blood pressure of < 130/80 mmHg. Patients with proteinuria (> 1 g/24 hours) benefit from even more aggressive blood pressure control (< 125/75 mmHg) in terms of slowing progression of kidney disease.

First-line therapy should comprise lifestyle changes, such as reducing salt intake, moderating alcohol intake, stopping smoking and taking regular exercise. Virtually all patients require an ACE inhibitor or an ARB as first-line therapy (Figure 5.2). Usually, more than one drug is required, and a β-blocker, a calcium-channel blocker or a diuretic agent can be added. The key features of several commonly used antihypertensive drug classes are shown in Table 5.2. The choice of drugs can be influenced by comorbid conditions, as shown in Table 5.3.

Most recent studies (such as the Antihypertensive and Lipid-Lowering Treatment to Prevent Heart Attack Trial, ALLHAT) have shown that achieving optimal blood pressure goals requires multiple drugs, that control of blood pressure using a stepped approach can take up to 2 years and that, in simple essential hypertension, the newer, more expensive drugs do not offer great benefits over thiazide diuretics.

Renovascular disease is a remediable form of hypertension and should be excluded in high-risk patients, such as elderly hypertensives with evidence of diffuse atherosclerosis, in refractory or malignant hypertension, in those with 'flash' pulmonary edema and in individuals with an abdominal bruit. In young women with hypertension of recent

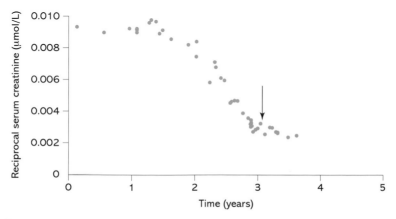

Figure 5.2 Reciprocal creatinine plot showing how treatment with angiotensin-converting-enzyme inhibitor slows the rate of decline in renal function (arrow).

TABLE 5.2

Key features of commonly used classes of antihypertensive drugs

Angiotensin-converting-enzyme inhibitors

- Renoprotective in chronic kidney disease
- Cardioprotective
- Antiproteinuric
- Generally well tolerated (cough 10–15%, angioedema 0.3%)

Angiotensin-receptor blockers

- Renoprotective in chronic kidney disease
- Cardioprotective
- Antiproteinuric
- Generally well tolerated

β-blockers

- Lower morbidity and mortality after myocardial infarction
- Potentially diabetogenic
- May mask hypoglycemia
- Lowers high-density lipoprotein cholesterol and raises triglyceride levels

Calcium-channel blockers

- Efficacious in multiple settings (blacks, diabetics, elderly)
- Useful in diastolic dysfunction
- Combination with β-blockers can result in severe bradycardia

Diuretics

- Preferred agent in congestive heart failure
- Inexpensive
- Associated hypokalemia, lipid abnormalities
- Increased risk of overt diabetes among patients with impaired glucose tolerance (thiazides)

α-blockers

- Useful in men with prostatic hypertrophy
- Metabolically neutral

TABLE 5.3

High-risk comorbid conditions and recommended treatment

Comorbid condition	Recommended treatment				
	Diuretic	β-blocker	ACE inhibitor	ARB	Calcium-channel blocker
Heart failure	+	+	+	+	+
Post-myocardial infarction		+	+	+	
Coronary artery disease		+	+	+	
Diabetes	+	+	+	+	
Chronic kidney disease			+	+	+

ACE, angiotensin-converting enzyme; ARB, angiotensin-receptor blocker.

onset, fibromuscular renal-artery disease should be excluded. The preferred diagnostic tests include magnetic resonance angiography and ACE-inhibitor renography. Duplex ultrasonography with Doppler flow measurements can be a useful screening test. The definitive diagnostic tests in almost all patients are still digital subtraction angiography or arteriography (Figure 5.3), but both carry a risk of contrast nephropathy and cholesterol embolization.

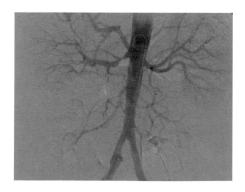

Figure 5.3 Digital subtraction angiogram showing right renal artery stenosis.

Angioplasty (with or without stenting) does not benefit all patients, as many have diffuse vascular disease including intrarenal blood vessels, and intervention carries risks (see above). Patients unlikely to have a positive response (and perhaps all patients) should receive aggressive medical therapy to control blood pressure, together with statins and aspirin. Surgery to bypass the stenotic lesion is now reserved for lesions that cannot be treated by angioplasty.

Hypertensive emergencies are situations in which an immediate reduction in blood pressure is required in order to prevent or treat acute progressive target organ damage. In such cases, a thorough history and physical examination should be undertaken (Table 5.4), which should include fundoscopy and urine tests for hematuria, proteinuria and red-cell casts. Other investigations should include tests for microangiopathic hemolytic anemia with red-cell fragmentation, renal dysfunction, evidence of left ventricular hypertrophy and strain, and ischemia on electrocardiography and echocardiography.

The management of a hypertensive emergency requires immediate hospitalization, usually in an intensive care unit, with arterial blood pressure monitoring, central vein catheterization and, occasionally, the use of parenteral drugs such as nitroprusside, glyceryl trinitrate, hydralazine, labetalol or fenoldopam (this last not licensed in the UK). Parenteral drugs are rarely needed, since blood pressure can usually be

TABLE 5.4

Clinical features associated with a hypertensive emergency

- Severe rise in blood pressure (diastolic pressure > 140 mmHg)
- Fundoscopy shows hemorrhages, exudates and papilledema
- Acute renal failure with proteinuria, hematuria and red-cell casts on urinalysis
- Encephalopathy, headaches, confusion, delirium, visual defects, seizures and coma
- Microangiopathic hemolytic anemia
- Nausea and vomiting

controlled with oral agents such as captopril (fast acting), labetalol (both α- and β-blockade) and clonidine.

Pregnancy. Hypertension in pregnancy is discussed in Chapter 12.

Diabetic nephropathy

Diabetic nephropathy is the most common cause of ESRF in Europe and the USA. Its prevalence is increasing as diabetic patients are living longer and the complications of diabetes are better controlled, and also because those who require renal replacement therapy are now accepted onto dialysis programs from which they had previously been excluded. There is considerable racial/ethnic variability in the incidence of diabetes. In the USA diabetes, and thus ESRF, is more common among native Americans, Hispanics (especially Mexican-Americans), African-Americans, Asian Indians and South Asians (Figure 5.4). ESRF secondary to diabetes mellitus is seen in 45% of patients in the USA, compared with 15% in the UK.

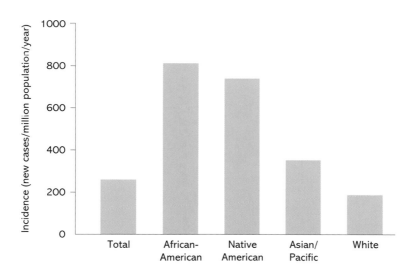

Figure 5.4 Incidence of end-stage renal failure (ESRF) in the USA according to racial background (adjusted for age and sex). In the UK, South Asians have a similar excess of ESRF over whites. The excess is mostly due to diabetes.

Diabetic nephropathy is defined by the presence of proteinuria; overt nephropathy is characterized by albuminuria of more than 300 mg/24 hours or 200 µg/minute, and renal dysfunction with a progressive decline in kidney function over time and hypertension may be present. The pathology of nephropathy in type 1 and type 2 diabetes is identical and comprises glomerular hypertrophy, glomerular basement membrane thickening, mesangial matrix accumulation and nodular glomerulosclerosis (Figure 5.5).

Natural history (Table 5.5). The earliest clinical evidence of nephropathy is the appearance of microalbuminuria, which is a low but abnormal amount of albumin in the urine (> 30 mg/24 hours or 20 µg/minute). Microalbuminuria can also be detected by an increased albumin:creatinine ratio in a spot urine sample (> 2.5 mg/mmol in men or 3.5 mg/mmol in women), which avoids the need for timed urine collections. Patients with early disease have incipient nephropathy and without specific interventions may progress to overt or clinical albuminuria over a period of 2–10 years. Most patients will also develop hypertension, which initially manifests as the absence of a

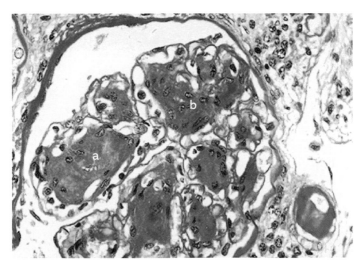

Figure 5.5 High-power photomicrograph of a glomerulus from a patient with diabetic kidney disease showing (a) mesangial matrix accumulation and (b) Kimmelstiel–Wilson nodules.

TABLE 5.5

Clinical features of diabetic kidney disease by stage

Stage 1

Early, predominantly physiological changes such as hyperfiltration (GFR supernormal)

Stage 2

Progressive thickening of glomerular basement membrane, mesangial matrix accumulation, glomerular hypertrophy; GFR remains in normal range and proteinuria is not present

Stage 3

Microalbuminuria (30–300 mg/24 hours, urine albumin:creatinine ratio > 2.5 mg/mmol creatinine in men or 3.5 mg/mmol in women) with associated hypertension

Stage 4

Overt nephropathy – urine albumin ≥ 300 mg/24 hours or albumin:creatinine ratio > 30 mg/mmol, with systolic hypertension, reduced GFR, continued structural changes, and evidence of glomerular sclerosis and arteriolar hyalinosis

Stage 5

Extensively scarred kidney; patient either in or near end-stage renal failure

GFR, glomerular filtration rate.

nocturnal dip in blood pressure, but later becomes sustained hypertension.

The degree of albuminuria varies quite significantly, but not uncommonly reaches nephrotic levels (> 3.5 g/24 hours). Once clinical albuminuria has developed, the GFR often declines relentlessly by 5–15 mL/minute/year. The mortality of patients with diabetic nephropathy is higher than in other patients because of a 4–8-fold increase in the rate of cardiovascular complications. In patients with both type 1 and type 2 diabetes, the onset of microalbuminuria is a major risk factor for both cardiovascular disease and mortality, and is also associated with retinopathy, left ventricular cardiac dysfunction and dyslipidemia, as well as hypertension. In all patients with microalbuminuria, other cardiovascular risk factors should be managed by, for example, lowering low-density lipoprotein (LDL) cholesterol, the use of antihypertensive therapy, cessation of smoking and taking exercise.

Screening for diabetic nephropathy

Methods. Four methods of screening for microalbuminuria are available (Table 5.6). A definitive diagnosis of microalbuminuria requires a positive result from at least two of three samples within a 3–6-month period, because of high day-to-day variability in urine albumin excretion. Screening dipsticks for microalbumin have acceptable sensitivity (95%) and specificity (93%) when used by trained personnel. All positive tests using reagent strips should be confirmed by more specific methods.

TABLE 5.6

Methods of measuring albumin excretion

Method	Advantages	Disadvantages
Urinalysis by microalbumin dipstick	Simple, cheap, rapid	Non-quantitative, small false-negative rate, does not correct for urine concentration
Albumin:creatinine ratio in a random spot urine collection	Simple, cheap, quantitative	Morning urine collection preferred because of the known diurnal variation in albumin excretion
24-hour or timed urine collection with measurement of albumin and creatinine	Accurate, inexpensive, quantitative, simultaneous assessment of renal function by measuring creatinine clearance	Urine collection often incomplete, high non-compliance rate, requires simultaneous measurement of serum creatinine (for creatinine clearance)
Specific immunoassays for urinary albumin	Rapid, simple, portable	Not standardized, expensive

Type 2 diabetes. All patients with type 2 diabetes should be screened for incipient or established diabetic nephropathy, because microalbuminuria is present at diagnosis in approximately 25% of patients. If urinalysis is positive for protein (in the absence of infection), it is very likely that the patient has clinical albuminuria (> 300 mg/24 hours), which has important implications in terms of the progression of renal disease and overall cardiovascular risks. Positive urinalysis should be confirmed quantitatively (e.g. spot urine albumin:creatinine ratio), and patients in whom urinalysis is negative for protein require quantitative assessment for microalbuminuria.

Type 1 diabetes. In contrast, microalbuminuria is rarely present at the time of diagnosis of type 1 diabetes or before puberty, and therefore screening should begin with the onset of puberty or 5 years after the diagnosis and be performed annually.

Risk factors. The major factor influencing the development of diabetic nephropathy is hyperglycemia. Persistent hyperglycemia leads to the development of glycosylated macromolecules and their conversion to advanced glycosylation end products. This process results in thickening of the basement membranes (including the glomerular basement membrane) and accumulation of matrix proteins within the glomeruli.

Although genetic factors predispose individuals to develop diabetes, whether they also influence the rate of progression of the nephropathy remains controversial. The racial and familial distribution of diabetes also suggests a role for as yet undetermined polygenic influences. Other risk factors include male gender and smoking. Apart from glycemic control, the other major factor determining progression through diabetic nephropathy is hypertension (see below).

Prevention and treatment. Aggressive intervention in patients with either incipient or established nephropathy has been shown unequivocally to prevent progression of kidney disease. Strategies include aggressive glycemic control, angiotensin blockade, control of blood pressure, protein restriction and smoking cessation (Figure 5.6 and Table 5.7).

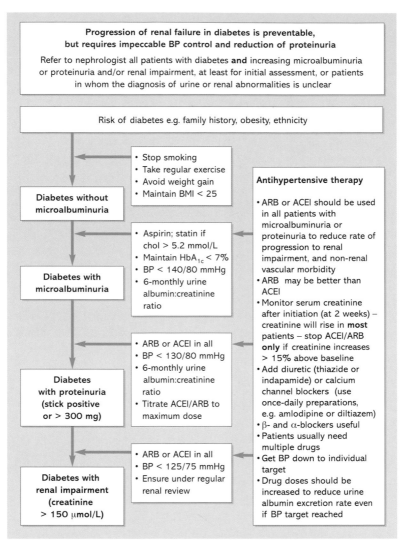

Figure 5.6 Flow chart for the prevention and treatment of diabetic nephropathy in a community setting. All patients with diabetes *and* increasing microalbuminuria or proteinuria and/or renal impairment should be referred to a nephrologist, at least for initial assessment, as should patients in whom the diagnosis of urine or renal abnormalities is unclear. Progression of renal failure in diabetes is preventable and requires impeccable blood pressure control and reduction of proteinuria. ACEI, angiotensin-converting-enzyme inhibitor; ARB, angiotensin-receptor blocker; BP, blood pressure; chol, cholesterol.

TABLE 5.7

Management strategies in diabetic nephropathy

Target	Treatment
Blood pressure < 125/75 mmHg	Angiotensin-converting-enzyme inhibitors or angiotensin-receptor blockers in all patients; most patients need at least two or three drugs, including a diuretic, a calcium antagonist and an α-blocker or β-blocker with the choice of drug tailored to other comorbidities (e.g. β-blocker in angina, α-blocker in prostatism)
Glycosylated hemoglobin < 7%	May need to start insulin; metformin should be discontinued in progressive renal failure when creatinine > 200 μmol/L
Total cholesterol < 5 mmol/L (200 mg/dL) and low-density lipoprotein cholesterol < 3 mmol/L (130 mg/dL)	All patients with diabetes and renal disease should be managed as if they need secondary prevention for cardiovascular disease and not primary prevention; statins should be started early, and treatment to lower triglycerides may also be required
Smoking cessation	Advice and appropriate assistance
Obesity	Weight loss and regular exercise
Overall cardiovascular risk	Antioxidant vitamins (C and E) may be helpful
Diet	Fairly low protein, low saturated fat, low salt, and high fruit and vegetables (if not hyperkalemic)

The US Diabetes Control and Complications Trial (DCCT) and the UK Prospective Diabetes Study (UKPDS) have clearly shown that intensive therapy can significantly reduce the risk of the development of microalbuminuria and overt nephropathy in individuals with diabetes. In the UKPDS, there was a 75% reduction in the relative risk of doubling serum creatinine over 12 years.

Hypertension. Overwhelming evidence implicates hypertension as a major risk factor in the progression of diabetic nephropathy.

Hypertension usually appears during the microalbuminuric phase of disease although, in type 2 diabetes, it may result from other causes, such as renovascular disease. Both systolic and diastolic hypertension accelerate the progression of diabetic nephropathy. Aggressive management of hypertension reduces the progression of diabetic kidney disease. The VIIth report of the Joint National Committee on the Prevention, Detection, Evaluation and Treatment of High Blood Pressure recommends a target blood pressure in diabetics with kidney disease of 130/80 mmHg or lower. Angiotensin blockade should be the first-line therapy, but most patients will require multiple drugs.

The important role of angiotensin blockade in retarding the progression of both type 1 and 2 diabetic nephropathy is now well established. The use of either ACE inhibitors or ARBs should be integrated into the overall antihypertensive management strategy. In addition to reducing systemic blood pressure, angiotensin blockade reduces intraglomerular pressure, thereby protecting the nephron from ongoing damage, and has effects independent of lowering blood pressure. Many studies have shown that in diabetic (and non-diabetic) patients with kidney disease, angiotensin blockade can reduce the level of albuminuria and the rate of progression of renal disease to a greater degree than other antihypertensive agent.

The use of angiotensin blockers may, however, exacerbate hyperkalemia in patients with advanced renal insufficiency and/or hyporeninemic hypoaldosteronism (type IV renal tubular acidosis). Patients with bilateral renal artery stenosis and those with advanced renal disease, who are being treated concurrently with NSAIDs or who are volume depleted, may experience a rapid decline in renal function when started on an ACE inhibitor; it is likely that ARBs have a similar effect. This is usually reversible when the drug is discontinued.

As a high proportion of patients progress from microalbuminuria to overt nephropathy and subsequently to ESRF, ACE inhibitors or ARBs are recommended for all patients with microalbuminuria. The effect of an ACE inhibitor appears to be a class effect, so the choice of agent may depend on cost and compliance issues; the same is probably true for ARBs. There is increasing evidence that the use of both types of drug in combination is safe and effective.

Protein restriction has been shown to be effective in retarding progression of renal disease in several animal models by reducing glomerular hyperfiltration and intraglomerular pressures. While small studies in humans with diabetic nephropathy have shown that protein restriction (0.6 g/kg/day) confers a moderate benefit in retarding progression, restricting protein in diabetics is hard to achieve and may lead to protein malnutrition. Nevertheless, the general consensus is to prescribe a protein intake of approximately the adult recommended dietary allowance of 0.8 g/kg/day (10% of daily calories) in patients with overt nephropathy.

Key points – hypertension and diabetic nephropathy

- Hypertension is both an important cause and a consequence of renal disease.
- Blood pressure targets are low (< 130/80 mmHg or lower) in the presence of renal disease or diabetes.
- Multiple drugs are needed in almost all patients.
- Diabetic kidney disease should be treated at an early stage with angiotensin blockade.

Key references

Berl T, Hunsicker LG, Lewis JB et al. Cardiovascular outcomes in the Irbesartan Diabetic Nephropathy Trial of patients with type 2 diabetes and overt nephropathy. *Ann Intern Med* 2003;138:542–9.

Goals of antihypertensive therapy in CKD. *Am J Kidney Dis* 2004; 43(suppl 1): 65–230.

Sever PS, Dahlof B, Poulter NR et al. Prevention of coronary and stroke events with atorvastatin in hypertensive patients who have average or lower-than-average cholesterol concentrations, in the Anglo-Scandinavian Cardiac Outcomes Trial--Lipid Lowering Arm (ASCOT-LLA): a multicentre randomised controlled trial. *Lancet.* 2003;361:1149–58.

www.kidney.org/professionals/kdoqi/index.cfm

Glomerulonephritis is the term used to describe abnormalities of the glomerulus resulting from a variety of immune and inflammatory mechanisms. Glomerulonephritis is often described as primary, when there is no associated disease elsewhere, or secondary, when glomerular involvement is part of a systemic disease. This chapter considers primary glomerulonephritis; secondary glomerulonephritis is discussed in the context of systemic disease in Chapter 7.

Primary glomerulonephritis may be described or classified according to the clinical syndrome produced (e.g. nephrotic syndrome), the histopathologic appearance (e.g. membranous nephropathy) or the underlying etiology (relevant mainly in secondary causes). Unfortunately, there is no direct correlation between the clinical syndrome produced and the pathological description. In most glomerular diseases, the natural history and response to treatment have been defined with respect to the histopathologic diagnosis (except for nephrotic syndrome in children), so a pathological description is preferred when considering management.

Presentation

Glomerulonephritis presents in a limited number of ways, depending on the nature and severity of the glomerular injury.

- Mild disease can present with asymptomatic hematuria and/or proteinuria. If proteinuria becomes heavy, leading to hypoalbuminemia and fluid retention, it is described as the nephrotic syndrome.
- More severe, acute forms of glomerulonephritis may present with 'acute nephritic syndrome', which involves hematuria (sometimes macroscopic), proteinuria, a fall in GFR, salt and water retention, and hypertension.
- Rapidly progressive glomerulonephritis describes a rapid loss of renal function, such that the patient will be in ESRF within weeks or months.

- Chronic glomerulonephritis involves a much slower deterioration in renal function, usually over several years, accompanied by hematuria, proteinuria and hypertension.

Hypertension may also be the presenting feature of some forms of glomerulonephritis.

Pathological classification

Except in the mildest cases, or in nephrotic syndrome in children, the suspicion of glomerulonephritis should lead to renal biopsy. Although the commonly used pathological classification depends on light microscopy, immunohistochemistry and electron microscopy provide additional information and may give clues as to the etiology. A single glomerulus is depicted in Figure 6.1.

Histological patterns

Minimal change disease. Light microscopy is virtually normal, but there is widespread fusion of the epithelial cell foot processes on the

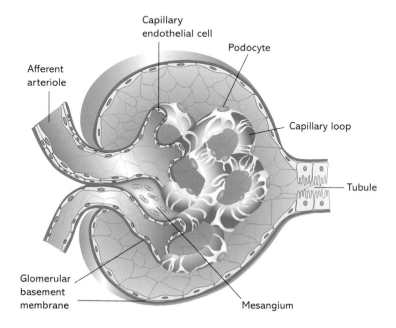

Figure 6.1 Structure of a single glomerulus.

outside of the glomerular basement membrane. Immunofluorescence is generally negative.

Focal segmental glomerulosclerosis. Some of the glomeruli show segmental scarring, together with foot process fusion as in minimal change disease.

Membranous nephropathy. Widespread thickening of the glomerular basement membrane occurs. Immunofluorescence reveals granular deposits of immunoglobulin and complement.

Mesangiocapillary glomerulonephritis (MCGN) is also known as membranoproliferative glomerulonephritis. There is proliferation of mesangial cells, an increase in mesangial matrix and thickening of the glomerular basement membrane. MCGN can be subdivided according to the appearance on electron microscopy.

Mesangial proliferative nephritis. Mesangial cell proliferation combined with matrix expansion occurs. It is most often seen in the context of immunoglobulin (Ig) A deposition, when it is known as IgA nephropathy. Other immunoglobulins and complement components may also be present.

Diffuse proliferative glomerulonephritis. Widespread hypercellularity occurs, caused by both infiltrating inflammatory cells and proliferation of endothelial and mesangial cells. There is generally deposition of immunoglobulins and complement around the capillary loops.

Focal and segmental proliferative glomerulonephritis generally occurs secondary to systemic disease, which is discussed in Chapter 7. There is often associated segmental necrosis of the capillary loops, which is followed by crescent formation. The term crescentic glomerulonephritis is used when there is an accumulation of cells outside the capillary loops, but within Bowman's capsule.

Crescentic glomerulonephritis (Figure 6.2) may occur as part of the evolution of certain forms of primary glomerulonephritis (e.g. IgA nephropathy or mesangiocapillary glomerulonephritis), but is more often seen in conditions such as Goodpasture's syndrome and systemic vasculitis. A condition previously described as idiopathic crescentic glomerulonephritis is now recognized as generally being due to renal limited vasculitis. The immunofluorescence findings are most informative in the diagnosis of crescentic glomerulonephritis (Table 6.1).

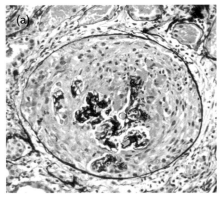

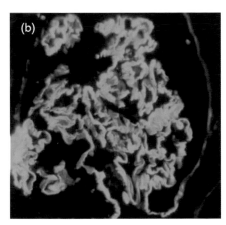

Figure 6.2 (a) Histological section of a renal biopsy showing a single glomerulus from a patient with rapidly progressive glomerulonephritis and antineutrophil cytoplasm antibody associated crescentic nephritis (the glomerulus is completely compressed by a crescent of cells).
(b) Immunohistology of renal biopsy showing antibody deposition on glomerular capillaries in anti-glomerular basement membrane disease (Goodpasture's syndrome).

TABLE 6.1

Classification of rapidly progressive glomerulonephritis based on immunofluorescence findings on renal biopsy

Immunofluorescence finding	Disorder
Linear deposits	Anti-glomerular basement membrane disease
Granular deposits	Primary or secondary immune complex glomerulonephritis
No (or few) deposits	Antineutrophil cytoplasm antibody-associated glomerulonephritis

Investigations

The investigations consists of an assessment of the severity of glomerular injury, together with a search for the cause (Table 6.2).

Clinical features and management

It is possible to provide only a brief outline here; further information should be sought from expert sources in order to manage patients.

TABLE 6.2

Investigation of glomerulonephritis

Investigation	Comment
Urine dipstick and microscopy	In glomerulonephritis, hematuria and/or proteinuria will be found and, in some forms, red-cell casts
Urine protein quantification	Measured in 24-hour urine sample or by protein:creatinine ratio
Glomerular filtration rate	Determined from serum creatinine and patient characteristics using a formula, or by 24-hour creatinine clearance
Biochemistry	Serum albumin low in nephrotic syndrome; high potassium, low bicarbonate and high phosphate in renal failure
Glucose	To exclude diabetes
Serum immunoglobulins, serum and urine protein electrophoresis	To exclude myeloma
Serum complement	Low in systemic lupus erythematosus and cryoglobulinemia and some forms of primary glomerulonephritis
Antineutrophil cytoplasm antibody, anti-glomerular basement membrane antibodies and antinuclear antibodies	Found in the associated disease

Minimal change disease accounts for most cases of nephrotic syndrome in children, and about 20% of cases in adults. It is associated with atopy in children and may be related to underlying Hodgkin's disease in adults. It usually responds to a course of high-dose prednisolone, but relapse is frequent. Relapsing disease may go into remission following treatment with prednisolone and cyclophosphamide. Alternatively, ciclosporin can be used, but relapses may occur when the drug is discontinued. Although severe nephrotic syndrome has its own complications (e.g. thrombotic episodes, infection), minimal change disease does not progress to ESRF.

Focal segmental glomerulosclerosis is a common cause of nephrotic syndrome in older children and younger adults; it may be associated with hematuria. About 50% of patients may respond to a course of high-dose prednisolone, although treatment for up to 4 months is often required in adults. If this is unsuccessful, some patients may respond to the addition of cyclophosphamide, and ciclosporin can be used to reduce proteinuria. Focal segmental glomerulosclerosis often progresses to ESRF over several years, but progression may be curtailed by treatment with corticosteroids.

A variant known as 'collapsing glomerulopathy' is associated with infection with human immunodeficiency virus (HIV). Antiretroviral therapy may be effective, and some patients respond to additional corticosteroids.

Membranous nephropathy is the most common cause of nephrotic syndrome in older adults. Hematuria is rare. Although many cases are idiopathic, it may also be secondary to SLE, hepatitis B, malignancy, or the use of gold or penicillamine. The idiopathic form may respond to a treatment regimen involving alternate months of corticosteroids and chlorambucil or cyclophosphamide (often known as the 'Ponticelli regimen'), or to ciclosporin. It progresses to ESRF in 30–50% of patients.

Mesangiocapillary glomerulonephritis is an uncommon disorder that can present as nephrotic syndrome or nephritic syndrome in children and young adults. Secondary forms of the disease are associated with hepatitis C with or without cryoglobulins, other chronic infections and SLE. Despite the lack of evidence from controlled studies, nephrotic patients with primary MCGN are often treated with corticosteroids.

IgA nephropathy is the most common form of glomerulonephritis worldwide. It often presents with macroscopic hematuria, which may be precipitated within a few days by an upper respiratory tract infection. It is also detected as asymptomatic hematuria and/or proteinuria, and can present with nephrotic syndrome. Some studies suggest that a course of high-dose prednisolone can reduce proteinuria and delay renal impairment. In patients with deteriorating renal function, the addition of immunosuppressive drugs has been proposed. There are conflicting reports of the benefit of high-dose fish oil, but one US study suggests slowing of renal impairment. Although progression is slow, 20–30% of patients may eventually develop ESRF. The renal lesion of Henoch–Schönlein purpura is similar to that of IgA nephropathy, and this may be a variant of the same disease.

Diffuse proliferative glomerulonephritis generally presents with an acute nephritic syndrome two or more weeks after an infection. Classically, the disease is caused by streptococcal infection, either of the pharynx or the skin. Although rare in developed countries, poststreptococcal glomerulonephritis remains common in the developing world. Many other bacterial and viral causes have now been described. Almost all children will recover without treatment (other than antibiotics for the infection), but a small proportion of adults may develop renal impairment.

Crescentic glomerulonephritis should be treated according to the underlying cause. So-called idiopathic crescentic glomerulonephritis is now widely regarded as a form of antineutrophil cytoplasm antibody (ANCA)-positive vasculitis limited to the kidney. It presents with the clinical syndrome of rapidly progressive glomerulonephritis. Without treatment, the disease progresses to ESRF within a few weeks or months, but prednisolone and cyclophosphamide are generally effective in patients before severe renal damage occurs. The addition of plasma exchange or pulse doses of methylprednisolone is recommended in patients with advanced renal disease. Recent evidence suggests that plasma exchange may be the more effective approach.

Goodpasture's syndrome is due to autoantibodies directed against the α3 chain of type IV collagen, which is a major structural component of the glomerular basement membrane. This collagen is also found in the alveolar basement membrane and accounts for the pulmonary hemorrhage that is seen in 50% of patients with this disorder (Figure 6.3).

The syndrome presents with rapidly progressive glomerulonephritis, usually leading to renal failure within 6 months if untreated. Treatment with prednisolone and cyclophosphamide, combined with plasma exchange to remove circulating anti-glomerular basement membrane antibodies rapidly, is generally effective if started before renal disease is advanced. However, patients will seldom recover renal function once they start dialysis. It is extremely rare for patients to relapse, and the long-term outcome is good following successful treatment.

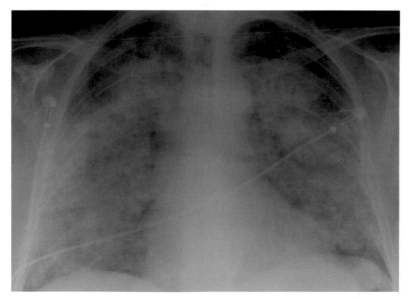

Figure 6.3 Chest radiograph showing extensive pulmonary hemorrhage in a patient with Goodpasture's syndrome.

Key points – glomerulonephritis

- Glomerulonephritis should be considered in all patients with urine abnormalities.
- Urgent investigations are needed to determine the precise type.
- Treatments are available for most categories of glomerulonephritis.
- Crescentic glomerulonephritis requires urgent and aggressive immunosuppression.

Key reference

Levy JB, Pusey CD. Crescentic glomerulonephritis. In: Brady HR, Wilcox CS, eds. *Therapy in Nephrology and Hypertension*, 2nd edn. Philadelphia: WB Saunders, 2003.

7 Systemic disease

Glomerular or tubular involvement may be a major feature of systemic autoimmune diseases, and may result from the deposition of abnormal proteins in dysproteinemias. Diabetic nephropathy is becoming the commonest cause of renal failure in developed countries; this is discussed in Chapter 5.

Systemic lupus erythematosus

SLE is a multisystem autoimmune disease that is most common in young women and often affects the joints, skin, nervous system and kidneys. Most patients with SLE will eventually develop kidney disease. This may affect the glomeruli directly, small blood vessels within the kidney or the interstitium. A variety of forms of lupus nephritis can be identified by standard light microscopy (Table 7.1). In classes I and II, mesangial deposits of immunoglobulin with or without complement are found. In classes III and IV, there is widespread deposition of various classes of immunoglobulin and complement along the capillary walls. In class V, subepithelial deposits predominate, as in primary membranous nephropathy.

Clinical features. Lupus nephritis can present with any of the clinical syndromes described earlier, depending on the severity of glomerular injury. Serology will often show elevated levels of anti-DNA antibodies and anti-C1q antibodies, together with reduced levels of serum complement C4 and/or C3. The erythrocyte sedimentation rate (ESR) is often raised, but the C-reactive protein may be normal unless an accompanying infection is present.

Treatment depends on the severity of the renal lesion. There is good evidence for using a combination of prednisolone and pulsed cyclophosphamide in class III and IV lupus nephritis. Recent studies suggest that mycophenolate mofetil, together with prednisolone, is also effective. Since the disease runs a relapsing and remitting course,

TABLE 7.1

New classification of lupus nephritis

Class I

- Minimal mesangial lupus nephritis

Class II

- Mesangial proliferative lupus nephritis

Class III

- Focal lupus nephritis

Class IV

- Class IV-S – diffuse segmental lupus nephritis
- Class IV-G – global lupus nephritis

Class V

- Membranous lupus nephritis

Class VI

- Advanced sclerosing lupus nephritis

Source: Weening JJ, D'Agati VD, Schwartz MM et al. The classification of glomerulonephritis in systemic lupus erythematosus revisited. *Kidney Int* 2004;65:521–30. Reproduced with permission of Blackwell Publishing.

maintenance therapy, often with low-dose prednisolone and azathioprine, is generally required.

Primary systemic vasculitis

Primary vasculitides cause necrotizing inflammation of the blood vessels, and can be classified according to the size of blood vessel they affect (Figure 7.1).

Primary vasculitides affecting small blood vessels, which include Wegener's granulomatosis, microscopic polyangiitis and, less commonly, Churg–Strauss syndrome, often cause glomerulonephritis. In some patients, vasculitis appears to be restricted to the kidney. These disorders show a slight male predominance and are more common in

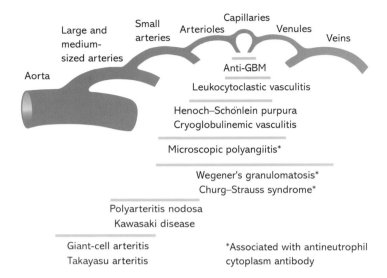

Figure 7.1 Classification of systemic vasculitis. GBM, glomerular basement membrane.

the elderly. The characteristic glomerular lesion is a focal and segmental necrotizing glomerulonephritis, which often progresses to crescent formation. There are no or scanty immune deposits.

Clinical features. Patients generally present with a rapidly progressive glomerulonephritis, although in some patients, there may be repeated episodes of less severe renal disease, leading to glomerular scarring together with active lesions. ANCAs have a high sensitivity and specificity in the diagnosis of these diseases, and can be divided according to the pattern seen on human neutrophils by immunofluorescence (Figure 7.2). Cytoplasmic ANCAs (cANCAs; Figure 7.2a) are usually the result of reactivity against proteinase 3, and are most often associated with Wegener's granulomatosis. Perinuclear ANCAs (pANCAs; Figure 7.2b) are often associated with reactivity against myeloperoxidase, and are more commonly seen in microscopic polyangiitis and renal limited vasculitis.

Treatment. Most patients respond well to treatment with prednisolone and cyclophosphamide. Once remission has been induced (generally by

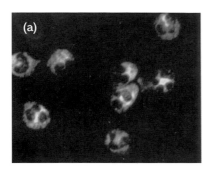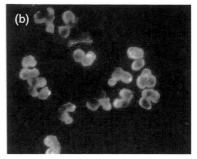

Figure 7.2 Antineutrophil cytoplasm antibody (ANCA) as shown by immuno-fluorescence using neutrophils. (a) Cytoplasmic ANCA; (b) perinuclear ANCA.

3 months), cyclophosphamide may be replaced by azathioprine for maintenance therapy. Patients with severe renal failure or other life-threatening features of disease are generally treated with additional intravenous methylprednisolone and/or plasma exchange. There is recent evidence that plasma exchange may be more effective than methylprednisolone in salvaging renal function in patients with advanced renal failure. With aggressive treatment, most patients, even those on dialysis, will recover renal function.

Hemolytic uremic syndrome

HUS is a form of thrombotic microangiopathy, with a tendency to affect the kidney. Renal histology reveals widespread intraglomerular thrombi, together with an occlusive vasculopathy. Renal involvement is often accompanied by hematologic and neurological manifestations. There is some clinical overlap with thrombotic thrombocytopenic purpura (TTP), though different disease mechanisms are involved.

Children. HUS in children is commonly related to gastrointestinal infection with *Escherichia coli* O157, which produces a verotoxin thought to damage endothelial cells. Most affected children will recover spontaneously, though some are left with renal impairment. The role of specific treatment in this so-called D+ HUS is unclear.

Adults may develop HUS sporadically (without obvious infection), on a familial basis or related to a variety of drugs. Some adults with HUS have been shown to have deficiencies in complement regulatory proteins, such as factor H. The principle of treatment is to replace deficient plasma components, together with the removal of potentially harmful abnormal components. This is achieved by plasma exchange with fresh frozen plasma, often accompanied by corticosteroids to reduce inflammation. No good trials of treatment have been reported in HUS, though plasma exchange with fresh frozen plasma has been shown to be effective in TTP.

Systemic sclerosis

Systemic sclerosis may affect the kidney by causing an obstructive vasculopathy of small renal arteries – so-called 'scleroderma kidney'.

Clinical features. Systemic sclerosis of the kidney presents with subacute or acute renal impairment. Renal failure may be compounded by vasospasm in addition to the structural lesions. Although systemic features of scleroderma are generally present (e.g. thickening of the skin, telangiectasia, esophageal dysfunction), renal involvement may occasionally be the presenting feature.

Treatment with ACE inhibitors improves the renal outcome. Prostacyclin may relieve spasm of intrarenal arteries.

Sarcoidosis

Sarcoidosis is a disease of unknown etiology, characterized by granulomatous inflammation of a number of organs, including the lungs and kidneys. The typical renal lesion is a granulomatous tubulointerstitial nephritis, which can lead to renal impairment. This will generally respond to treatment with corticosteroids. Sarcoidosis may also lead to hypercalcemia, which can itself cause renal dysfunction.

Cryoglobulinemia

Cryoglobulins are immunoglobulins that precipitate in the cold; three major types have been described (Table 7.2). Type I cryoglobulins are more likely to result in renal damage through high viscosity or

TABLE 7.2

Classification of cryoglobulinemia

Cryoglobulin		Associated disease
Type I	Monoclonal, usually IgM, occasionally IgG, rarely IgA	Lymphoproliferative diseases (e.g. myeloma, Waldenström's macroglobulinemia, non-Hodgkin's lymphoma)
Type II	Mixture of monoclonal rheumatoid factor (usually IgM) and polyclonal Ig	Lymphoproliferative diseases; hepatitis C or rarely other chronic infections
Type III	Mixture of polyclonal rheumatoid factor and polyclonal Ig	Malignancy, chronic infections, autoimmune disease (e.g. systemic lupus erythematosus), chronic liver disease

Ig, immunoglobulin.

intravascular deposition. Treatment of acute renal disease in type I cryoglobulinemia generally involves plasma exchange to reduce paraprotein levels, together with appropriate chemotherapy.

Type II cryoglobulins often lead to mesangiocapillary glomerulonephritis. Clinical features commonly include a purpuric rash, arthralgia and peripheral neuropathy. Many cases are associated with hepatitis C infection, when treatment with appropriate antiviral drugs is recommended. Plasma exchange may be helpful in removing circulating cryoglobulins in the most severe disease, and can be combined with prednisolone and cyclophosphamide therapy. Type III cryoglobulins are generally related to an underlying autoimmune disease or chronic infection. They rarely cause severe renal disease. Treatment involves management of the underlying disorder.

Myeloma and monoclonal dysproteinemias

Multiple myeloma may affect the kidney in many different ways (Table 7.3). Cast nephropathy appears to be an increasingly common

TABLE 7.3

Causes of renal dysfunction in myeloma

- Light chain cast nephropathy
- Light and heavy chain deposition disease
- AL amyloidosis
- Cryoglobulinemia
- Hypercalcemic nephropathy
- Acute urate nephropathy
- Acute interstitial nephritis
- Pyelonephritis
- Obstructive uropathy

cause of ARF or subacute renal failure, particularly in the elderly. Adequate hydration and correction of hypercalcemia and other metabolic abnormalities are crucial. There is some evidence that plasma exchange (to reduce paraprotein levels) is beneficial, accompanied by chemotherapy to treat the myeloma (often vincristine, adriamycin and dexamethasone in younger adults).

Amyloidosis

The term amyloid is used to describe insoluble deposits of protein formed by the association of amyloid P component, together with other proteins that possess characteristic physicochemical properties. The commonest forms affecting the kidney are AL amyloid, in which Ig light chains are involved, and AA amyloid, in which amyloid A protein produced by chronic inflammation is involved. More rarely, mutations in other serum proteins can lead to amyloidosis of a familial nature (e.g. mutations in transthyretin, lysosyme, apolipoprotein E). Amyloid deposition in the kidney commonly results in nephrotic syndrome, usually associated with progressive renal impairment. Deposition in other organs depends on the type of amyloid, but there is commonly damage to the liver, spleen, heart and nervous system. Reducing the load of amyloid precursor proteins may allow resolution of the condition (slowly). This might be achieved by appropriate chemotherapy for dysproteinemia in AL amyloid, or by tight control of the underlying inflammatory disease in AA amyloid.

> **Key points – systemic disease**
>
> - Systemic lupus erythematosus commonly causes kidney disease, which can be very severe and requires immunosuppression.
> - Vasculitis is common in the elderly and can be successfully treated if diagnosed early.
> - Long-term treatment is usually needed for both vasculitis and systemic lupus erythematosus with kidney involvement.
> - Atheromatous renal vascular disease is very common and reflects widespread arterial pathology.

Atherosclerotic renovascular disease

Atherosclerotic renovascular disease is an increasingly important cause of established renal failure in the elderly. Atheroma of the renal arteries is commonly seen as an extension of aortic disease, so atheromatous renal artery stenosis is usually proximal (Figure 7.3).

The natural history is generally of progression. Atherosclerosis may lead to renal dysfunction by occlusion of the arterial lumen, though this requires a greater than 70% stenosis. Perhaps of greater importance, atheroma of the renal artery can lead to cholesterol embolization of intrarenal vessels or glomeruli, which often causes irreversible renal failure.

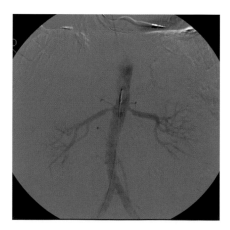

Figure 7.3 Bilateral renal artery stenosis and atheromatous aorta.

Radiological intervention using angioplasty, with or without stenting, is generally successful in relieving renal artery stenosis. Current indications for radiological intervention are summarized in Table 7.4. However, the long-term effects on renal function have not been adequately studied, and clinical trials are in progress.

TABLE 7.4

Indications for radiological intervention in atherosclerotic renovascular disease

Significant stenosis (> 60%) with:

- Resistant hypertension
- Flash pulmonary edema
- Renal impairment related to angiotensin-converting-enzyme inhibitors
- Progressively declining renal function
- Single functioning kidney

Key references

Flanc RS, Roberts MA, Strippoli GF et al. Treatment of diffuse proliferative lupus nephritis: a meta-analysis of randomized controlled trials. *Am J Kidney Dis* 2004;43:197–208.

Main J. When should atheromatous renal artery stenosis be considered? A guide for the general physician. *Clin Med* 2003;3:520–5.

Seo P, Stone JH. The antineutrophil cytoplasmic antibody-associated vasculitides. *Am J Med* 2004;117: 39–50.

Textor SC. Ischemic nephropathy: where are we now? *J Am Soc Nephrol* 2004;15:1974–82.

Autosomal-dominant polycystic kidney disease

Autosomal-dominant polycystic kidney disease (APKD) is a common inherited multisystem disease in which patients develop multiple bilateral renal cysts, cysts in other organs and non-cystic extrarenal manifestations (Figure 8.1).

Pathophysiology. Most patients (85–90%) have a mutation in the *PKD1* gene, which encodes the protein polycystin. Mutations in a second gene, *PKD2*, and an unidentified third gene, can also cause APKD. The precise function of the proteins encoded by *PKD1* and *PKD2* has not been clarified, though they are likely to play a role in cell–cell and cell–matrix interactions, and possibly as a transmembrane ion channel. Cysts arise from focal dilatation of the tubules.

Clinical features of APKD are summarized in Table 8.1. APKD affects about 1 in 1000 people, making it one of the commonest inherited diseases. It is a common cause of ESRF; however, progression is slow in most patients, and not inevitable.

Diagnosis. Cysts are easily identified by ultrasound examination. Cysts are not commonly seen in the fetus or in children. They are, however, found in a number of conditions other than APKD, such

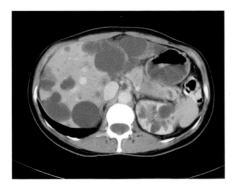

Figure 8.1 Computerized tomography scan showing polycystic kidneys and liver in autosomal-dominant polycystic kidney disease.

TABLE 8.1

Clinical features of autosomal-dominant polycystic kidney disease

Feature	Comment
Renal cyst formation	Causes pain, mass effects, gastrointestinal disturbance, cyst hemorrhage and hematuria
Urinary tract infection	Presents as cystitis, pyelonephritis, cyst infection or perinephric abscess; usually caused by Gram-negative organisms; mainly affects women
Renal stones	Occur in 20% of patients; usually uric acid or calcium oxalate
Hypertension	Found in 75% of patients before onset of renal failure; associated with renal size; significantly increases the risk of renal failure
Renal failure	50% of patients develop renal failure by the age of 50–70 years; earlier onset in those with *PKD1* mutations
Polycystic liver	Occurs in 25–70% of patients (increasing with increasing age); more common in women; causes symptoms from massive enlargement of liver or mass effect
Intracranial aneurysm	Occur in 8% patients, and family history common; screening not generally advised because aneurysms found are small, unlikely to rupture and require no treatment
Mitral valve prolapse	Common, but rarely significant

as simple cysts, tuberose sclerosis and von Hippel–Lindau disease. The absence of cysts in young people does not exclude the diagnosis, because they can form late in life, and screening of asymptomatic individuals is therefore not recommended before the age of 20 years. If negative, a scan should then be repeated at 5-yearly intervals in individuals with a family history. Genetic diagnosis by mutation analysis or linkage analysis is possible, but not always available, and may require blood samples from family members.

Treatment. No specific treatments are available. Pain may require strong analgesics, and nephrotoxic agents should be avoided. Cyst hemorrhage is usually self limiting. Upper tract infection should be treated with antibiotics that will penetrate cysts (fluoroquinolones). Stones are managed as in patients without APKD. Hypertension requires aggressive management, but should generally include an ACE inhibitor or ARBs. Liver cysts occasionally need resecting.

Hereditary nephritis (Alport's syndrome)

Hereditary nephritis is a group of rare genetic disorders that affects 2 in 100 000 people, and accounts for 3% of children and 0.2% of adults with ESRF in developed countries. It is caused by mutations in type IV collagen, which result in structurally defective glomerular (and other) basement membranes. Hereditary nephritis presents with hematuria and proteinuria, causes deafness and ocular changes, and, in a proportion of individuals, progresses to chronic renal failure, but with a wide variation in phenotype.

Pathophysiology. There are three genetic forms of hereditary nephritis:

- mutations in the *COL4A5* gene causing X-linked Alport's syndrome, which accounts for about 80% of patients
- mutations in either *COL4A3* or *COL4A4* causing autosomal-recessive disease, which accounts for about 15% of patients
- mutations causing autosomal-dominant inheritance, which are rare and account for only 5% of cases.

Clinical features. Hereditary nephritis has a variable clinical presentation (Table 8.2). Males invariably progress to ESRF, while females, despite hematuria, generally maintain renal function (15% may have renal insufficiency). Hematuria may be observed at birth. In adolescent boys, episodes of gross hematuria may be precipitated by upper respiratory infections. The absence of hematuria during the first 10 years of life makes it likely that a child will not be affected. The key pathological findings on renal biopsy are seen by electron microscopy (thickening of the glomerular basement membrane, lamellation and electron-lucent areas).

TABLE 8.2

Clinical features of hereditary nephritis

- Hematuria, proteinuria and hypertension
- Cochlear deafness
- Ocular abnormalities: anterior lenticonus and pigment changes in the perimacular region
- Platelet abnormalities (megathrombocytopenia)
- Prognosis: ESRD in all affected males with X-linked disease, benign course in affected females

Other organ involvement. About 50% of patients are deaf, males being more commonly affected than females. Deafness is usually progressive from birth onwards; in its early stages, the hearing deficit is detectable only by audiometry.

The most common ocular abnormalities are anterior lenticonus and/or pigment abnormalities of the macula. In lenticonus, the central portion of the lens protrudes into the anterior chamber, which causes progressive opacification of the lens leading to loss of visual acuity and progressive myopia. Lenticonus is usually associated with deafness and appears during the second to third decade of life. Pigment changes in the perimacular region consist of whitish or yellowish granulations surrounding the fovea. Hematologic defects (megathrombocytopenia) are rare.

Diagnosis. The differential diagnosis of hereditary nephritis includes various primary and secondary glomerular diseases causing hematuria, especially thin basement membrane disease and IgA nephropathy, and abnormalities of the urinary tract. The definitive diagnostic test is renal biopsy with electron microscopy, and immunohistology showing the absence of specific collagen proteins. Skin biopsy and immunohistology can also be used since the α3 collagen proteins are also found in the epidermal basement membrane.

Genetic analysis is the only reliable way to diagnose the carrier state in asymptomatic female members of affected families and to establish a

> **Key points – inherited kidney diseases**
>
> • Autosomal-dominant polycystic kidney disease is a common inherited disease.
> • Liver cysts are the commonest extrarenal manifestation.
> • Progression to end-stage renal failure is slow, and does not occur in all patients.
> • Alport's syndrome is an important but rare cause of hematuria.
> • Deafness and eye abnormalities are common in men with Alport's syndrome.

prenatal diagnosis. However, the clinical usefulness of molecular genetic analysis is limited; it is time consuming and expensive and only identifies 50% of mutations. Thus, the most common approach still focuses on making a histological diagnosis, followed by screening family members by urinalysis and genetic counseling.

Management. No specific treatments are available. Priorities are management of hypertension, slowing the progression of CKD and prevention of complications. Ultimately, chronic renal failure progresses to ESRF, requiring dialysis or transplantation. Transplant survival rates are similar to those for patients with other diagnoses. Anti-glomerular basement membrane nephritis involving the renal allograft may occur in a recipient with hereditary nephritis, because an immune response develops to a hitherto unseen type IV collagen antigen; however, this is rare and affects only 3–4% of male transplant recipients.

Surgical repair of cataracts or repair of the anterior lenticonus is possible. Loss of hearing is likely to be permanent. Young men with Alport's syndrome should use hearing protection in noisy environments.

Key references

Bogdanova N. Autosomal dominant polycystic kidney disease – clinical and genetic aspects. *Kidney Blood Press Res* 2002;25:265–83.

Gregory MC. Alport syndrome and thin basement membrane nephropathy: unraveling the tangled strands of type IV collagen. *Kidney Int* 2004;65:1109–10.

Urinary tract infection (UTI) is the presence of bacteria and white cells in the urine, together with symptoms; significant bacteriuria is defined as a urine culture yielding more than 10^5 colony-forming units (CFU) of bacteria per mL of urine. Cystitis is inflammation of the bladder, which is most commonly (but not only) caused by infection. UTI is the second most common infection after respiratory infection and, in the elderly, is the most common source of Gram-negative bacteremia. However, UTI is generally a disease of sexually active females; 1 in 3 women will develop a UTI during her lifetime, and 20% have a recurrence. UTI is a leading cause of morbidity and healthcare expenditure; in the USA alone, UTI accounts for approximately 7 million visits/year to primary care providers and more than 1 million hospitalizations, and costs the US healthcare system in excess of $1 billion/year.

Causes and risk factors

Most UTIs are caused by Gram-negative aerobic bacteria (Table 9.1). These bacteria are normally present in the colon and may enter the urethral opening from the skin around the anus and the vaginal introitus. Women may be more susceptible to UTI because their urethral opening is near the source of bacteria (i.e. anus, vagina) and their urethra is shorter, providing bacteria easier access to the bladder. In over 50% of patients, bacteria ascend further up the ureters to the kidneys.

Host factors predisposing to UTI are shown in Table 9.2. Factors influencing bacterial virulence are also important and include specific projecting hairlike structures called pili and fimbriae, which interact with the urothelium and enable the bacteria to adhere to the surface.

Sexual intercourse triggers UTI in some women for unknown reasons. Women who use a diaphragm develop infections more often, and condoms with spermicidal foam may allow the growth of E. coli in the vagina, which may enter the urethra. Urinary catheterization can

TABLE 9.1

Common causes of urinary tract infection

Source of infection	Organism	Incidence (%)
Community	Gram-negative	
	• *Escherichia coli*	80
	• *Klebsiella, Proteus, Enterobacter, Serratia*	10
	Gram-positive	
	• *Staphylococcus saprophyticus*	8
	• *Enterococci*	2
Hospital	Gram-negative	
	• *Escherichia coli*	50
	• *Klebsiella, Proteus, Enterobacter, Serratia*	40
	Gram-positive	
	• *Staphylococcus saprophyticus* and *S. aureus*	8
	• *Enterococcus faecalis*	2
	Yeasts	
	• *Candida, Blastomyces, Coccidiodes immitis*	< 5

TABLE 9.2

Host factors predisposing to urinary tract infection (UTI)

Premenopausal women	Postmenopausal women
• Sexual intercourse	• Previous UTI
• Spermicide cream	• Anatomic defects (e.g. incontinence, postvoid residual volume)
• Recent antibiotic use	
• Previous UTI	• Cystocele
• Maternal history of UTI	• Altered vaginal flora with estrogen deficiency

also cause UTIs by introducing bacteria into the urinary tract. In infants, bacteria from soiled diapers can enter the urethra and cause UTI. Other risk factors include bladder outlet obstruction (e.g. from kidney stones or benign prostatic hypertrophy), conditions that cause incomplete bladder emptying (e.g. spinal cord injury) and congenital abnormalities of the urinary tract (e.g. vesicoureteral reflux). In children less than 10 years of age, 30–50% of UTIs are associated with vesicoureteral reflux and renal scarring, which can lead to renal insufficiency if not treated.

Diagnosis

The diagnosis of UTI requires a good history, urinalysis (with a Gram stain if indicated) and a clean-catch urine specimen for culture and sensitivity testing (Table 9.3). Urine culture may be unnecessary in a woman with a convincing history and pyuria on dipstick analysis.

TABLE 9.3

Diagnosis of urinary tract infection

Technique	Feature identified
Urine dipstick	• Pyuria • Hematuria • Proteinuria
Urine sediment examination	• Leukocytes (upper limit of normal is 5 cells/high-power field) • Erythrocytes (upper limit of normal is 5 cells/high-power field) • Renal tubular epithelial cells • Bacteria, yeast • White-cell casts (suggestive of pyelonephritis)
Clean-catch urine for culture	• Positive culture
Imaging studies (ultrasound, radiograph of kidney, ureter and bladder or computerized tomography scan)	• Indicated in all children (together with a micturating cystourethrogram) • Indicated in men with complicated UTI • Indicated in women if response to treatment has been poor or recurrent episodes • Indicated for any UTI associated with bacteremia or pyelonephritis

Treatment

Most patients respond rapidly to therapy. Structural abnormalities, such as prostatic hypertrophy or renal calculi, require urologic referral. Hospitalization of patients with a UTI is unnecessary unless there is systemic toxicity and/or the patient requires intravenous antibiotic therapy. Measures such as drinking more fluid or cranberry juice, and alkalinization of urine with potassium citrate, are all unproven.

UTI syndromes

UTI may be either uncomplicated or complicated. Uncomplicated UTI occurs in healthy (usually) women in the community. Complicated UTI occurs because of the presence of an underlying anatomic, functional or pharmacological factor that predisposes to persistent or recurrent infection, or treatment failure (Table 9.4). About one-third of all UTIs are complicated. The different categories, criteria for diagnosis and treatment of both complicated and uncomplicated UTIs are summarized in Table 9.5.

Acute cystitis in young women is the most common category of UTI and occurs in young, sexually active women. Causative factors may include sexual activity itself and the use of diaphragms and spermicides. While traditionally the diagnosis of UTI is based on the presence of significant bacteriuria, one-third or more of symptomatic women with uncomplicated cystitis have less than 10^5 CFU/mL of urine, and a

TABLE 9.4

Clinical complications of urinary tract infection

- Hemorrhagic cystitis
- Abscess of the bladder wall (pyocystosis)
- Papillary necrosis
- Chronic pyelonephritis
- Renal abscess
- Renal failure
- Septic shock

TABLE 9.5

Urinary tract infections in adults

Diagnosis	Treatment

Acute uncomplicated cystitis

Clinical diagnosis or urine culture ($> 10^2$ CFU/mL)	• Treat for 3 days with: trimethoprim, trimethoprim–sulfamethoxazole, nitrofurantoin, ciprofloxacin (but should not be used as first-line agent)

Recurrent cystitis in young women

Urine culture ($> 10^2$–10^6 CFU/mL)	• Change contraception method • Treat as for acute uncomplicated cystitis • Consider prophylaxis for 6 months with: trimethoprim, 100 mg, trimethoprim–sulfamethoxazole, 480 mg, nitrofurantoin, 100 mg, norfloxacin, 200 mg

Postcoital urinary tract infection

History	• Consider single-dose, postcoital antibiotic prophylaxis using same drugs and doses as for recurrent cystitis prophylaxis as above

Acute cystitis in young men

Urine culture ($> 10^3$ CFU/mL)	• Treat for 7–14 days with trimethoprim, trimethoprim–sulfamethoxazole, nitrofurantoin or ciprofloxacin

Acute pyelonephritis

History and urine culture ($> 10^6$ CFU/mL)	• Treat for 7–14 days orally, or intravenously initially if unwell, with: ciprofloxacin, trimethoprim–sulfamethoxazole, gentamicin plus quinolone, third-generation cephalosporin, amoxicillin–clavulanic acid if Gram-positive organism

Asymptomatic bacteriuria in pregnancy

Urine culture ($> 10^5$ CFU/mL)	• Treat for 3–7 days with: amoxicillin, nitrofurantoin, cefalexin (avoid quinolones)

CONTINUED

TABLE 9.5 (CONTINUED)

Urinary tract infections in adults

Diagnosis	Treatment
Catheter-associated infection	
Urine culture ($> 10^5$ CFU/mL)	• Remove catheter if possible • Treat with antibiotics for 7–10 days according to sensitivity

CFU, colony-forming units.

convincing history with pyuria by dipstick has a high predictive value without the need for urine culture.

The symptoms of cystitis usually have a sudden onset and include urinary frequency, urgency and burning or painful voiding of small volumes of urine. Nocturia with suprapubic or low back pain is common. The urine is often turbid, and gross hematuria occurs in about 30% of patients. This is not a systemic infection, and patients should not be febrile or develop a raised ESR or C-reactive protein. Uncomplicated cystitis is most commonly caused by *F. coli* and is easily treated with antibiotics; 3-day courses may be better than single doses or 7-day courses (Table 9.5).

Recurrent cystitis in young women. Up to 20% of young women with acute cystitis develop recurrent UTIs. Hematuria and pyuria are almost always present. It is important to perform a urine culture to differentiate between relapse (infection with the same organism) and recurrence (infection with different organisms). Multiple infections caused by the same organism require longer courses of antibiotics and possibly further diagnostic tests (Table 9.5). In contrast, infections caused by different organisms are generally not associated with underlying anatomic abnormalities and do not require further investigation of the genitourinary tract. A negative urinalysis or Gram stain does not exclude cystitis in women with low bacterial counts.

Women who have more than three recurrences of UTI documented by urine culture within 1 year can be managed by either self-treatment of the acute episode, postcoital prophylaxis (if an association with sexual intercourse is established) or continuous daily prophylaxis (Table 9.5). This approach decreases the significant morbidity associated with recurrent UTIs and is not associated with induction of antibiotic resistance in the organisms. However, stopping antibiotic prophylaxis is associated with recurrence in over 50% of patients.

Acute cystitis in young men. UTI in men is most commonly associated with underlying urologic abnormalities. In younger men, however, UTI may result from unprotected anal intercourse, an uncircumcised penis, unprotected intercourse with a woman whose vagina is colonized with uropathogens and in those men with HIV infection and a CD4+ T-cell count below $200/\mu L$. The commonest urologic abnormalities that predispose to UTI are prostatic disease, outlet obstruction and urinary tract instrumentation.

A diagnosis of UTI can be made with a high degree of sensitivity and specificity if the patient has symptoms of UTI and bacteriuria of more than 10^3 CFU/mL of urine. Treatment should be given for a minimum of 7 days, and for as long as 6–12 weeks in acute prostatitis (Table 9.5). In complicated UTI, further diagnostic investigations should be performed, but no further action may be necessary in younger men who respond rapidly to treatment. Chronic prostatitis may be more occult and present only as recurrent bacteriuria, low-grade fever or back discomfort. It is the commonest cause of recurrent UTI in men.

Acute urethritis usually presents with dysuria and urethral discharge, and is caused by gonococci, *Chlamydia* or *Ureaplasma* (non-specific urethritis). It is often associated with vaginal discharge and dyspareunia. Midstream urine does not contain blood on urinalysis.

Urethral syndrome occurs in women complaining of recurrent dysuria and frequency, but with sterile urine or low bacterial counts that have not responded to antibiotics. Vaginitis is found in 30% of these women (*Candida*, *Trichomonas* or non-specific), but the cause is unknown in the remainder.

Acute pyelonephritis is bacterial infection of the kidney parenchyma. In men, pyelonephritis does not usually occur in the absence of underlying urologic abnormalities, whereas in women it may occur in association with, or as a consequence of, acute cystitis even in the absence of predisposing factors. Occasionally, bacterial infection is not ascending, but occurs by hematogenous spread of a virulent bacterial strain (e.g. *Salmonella*, *Staphylococcus aureus*). In some patients, pyelonephritis may present with mild cystitis-like symptoms accompanied by back pain, while in others, a more severe illness occurs characterized by fever, chills, hypotension and severe back pain with or without symptoms of acute cystitis.

In most cases, acute pyelonephritis is caused by specific uropathogenic strains of *E. coli* that possess adhesins. These strains are able to ascend the urinary tract and adhere to renal tubular cells. Patients have elevated C-reactive protein and white cell counts, pyuria and, in 20%, positive blood cultures. The urine may contain white-cell casts, but proteinuria is minimal. The commonest organisms are *E. coli*, staphylococci, enterococci, and *Klebsiella*. The differential diagnosis includes appendicitis, urolithiasis, pelvic inflammatory disease, ectopic pregnancy and ruptured ovarian cyst.

For patients with a mild presentation, oral therapy is sufficient (Table 9.5). For patients with more severe symptoms or with evidence of bacteremia, empiric parenteral antibiotic therapy is recommended for at least the first 1–3 days: a third-generation cephalosporin, aztreonam, a broad-spectrum penicillin, a quinolone, an aminoglycoside or trimethoprim–sulfamethoxazole, followed by oral therapy; in this case, treatment should be given for a minimum of 2 weeks.

Chronic pyelonephritis is a term usually reserved for recurrent episodes of pyelonephritis in the presence of vesicoureteric reflux in children, but can occur in other circumstances. Renal parenchymal scarring occurs and can lead to progressive renal failure.

Asymptomatic bacteriuria is bacteriuria of more than 10^5 CFU/mL of urine in asymptomatic individuals. Treatment is warranted only in certain circumstances (Table 9.6). Although up to 40% of the elderly

TABLE 9.6

Indications for treatment of asymptomatic bacteriuria

- Pregnancy, particularly in third trimester
- Predisposition to renal disease (e.g. polycystic kidney disease)
- Immunocompromised patient (e.g. renal transplant)
- Patients requiring urologic manipulation
- Patients with anatomic or urologic abnormalities of the urinary tract

have asymptomatic bacteriuria, it is unclear whether treatment is beneficial in reducing complications or mortality.

Between 2–10% of pregnancies are complicated by UTI; if left untreated, 25–30% of the women affected will develop pyelonephritis. Pregnancies that are complicated by pyelonephritis have been associated with low birth weight and premature infants. Thus, pregnant women should be screened for bacteriuria by urine culture at 12–16 weeks of gestation. Bacteriuria of more than 10^5 CFU/mL of urine is considered significant. Pregnant women with asymptomatic bacteriuria should be treated with a 3–7-day course of antibiotics, and the urine should subsequently be cultured to ensure cure and to avoid relapse. As *E. coli* is now commonly resistant to ampicillin, amoxicillin and cefalexin, treatment should be based on the results of susceptibility tests. Nitrofurantoin or trimethoprim–sulfamethoxazole may be used, but in the third trimester sulfonamides compete with bilirubin binding in the newborn.

Most pregnant women with pyelonephritis should be hospitalized. They should receive intravenous antibiotic therapy initially, then oral treatment for 14 days, followed by nightly suppressive therapy until delivery. Ceftriaxone is a suitable agent for inpatient treatment, but the fluoroquinolones should be avoided in pregnancy.

Catheter-associated urinary tract infection. The risk of bacteriuria is approximately 5%/day in patients with an indwelling urinary catheter. Therefore, bacteriuria is inevitable in patients undergoing long-term catheterization. Catheter-associated UTIs account for 40% of all nosocomial infections and are the most common source of Gram-negative bacteremia in hospitalized patients. The bacterial distribution reflects the nosocomial origin of the infections, which are often polymicrobial because many of the pathogens are acquired exogenously via manipulation of the catheter. Symptomatic bacteriuria in a patient with an indwelling catheter should be treated with antibiotics that cover potential nosocomial uropathogens. Patients with mild-to-moderate infections may be treated with an oral quinolone, usually for 10–14 days. Parenteral antibiotic therapy may be necessary for patients with severe infections or patients who are unable to tolerate oral medication. Treatment is not recommended for catheterized patients who have asymptomatic bacteriuria, with the exception of patients who are immunosuppressed after organ transplantation, patients at risk for bacterial endocarditis and patients who are about to undergo urinary tract instrumentation.

Key points – urinary tract infections

- Uncomplicated cystitis in women, diagnosed by history and pyuria, can be treated empirically with short courses of antibiotics.
- Recurrent cystitis in women may require longer courses or prophylactic antibiotics.
- Cystitis in men generally requires a formal urological assessment.
- Pyelonephritis usually requires intravenous antibiotics as initial treatment.

Key references

Car J. Recurrent urinary tract infection in women. *BMJ* 2003;327:1204.

Hooton T. The current management strategies for community-acquired urinary tract infection. *Infect Dis Clin North Am* 2003;17:303–32.

Kidney stones are a common cause of morbidity in the Western world, affecting 10–20% of the population during their lifetime and leading to hospitalization for 1 in 1000 of the general population each year. Over 80% of kidney stones occur in white men; they are much rarer in women and black people. The peak age of onset for kidney stone formation is 20–30 years, and the recurrence rate is high – up to 50% within 5 years.

There are four main types of kidney stones (Table 10.1).

- The most common stones contain calcium salts, and may be calcium oxalate, calcium phosphate or a mixture of both.
- Magnesium ammonium phosphate stones (struvite stones) mostly occur in association with an underlying urease-splitting bacterial infection of the urinary tract (e.g. *Proteus*). These stones often recur and are most often seen in patients with an associated anatomic abnormality.
- Pure uric acid stones usually occur in the context of hyperuricemia among patients with a gouty diathesis or a hematologic malignancy. Uric acid stones have a high recurrence rate.
- Cystine stones are extremely rare and occur in patients with

TABLE 10.1

Incidence of different types of kidney stone

Type of stone	Incidence (%)
Calcium	70–80
• calcium oxalate	70
• calcium phosphate	< 5
• mixed calcium oxalate/phosphate	< 5
Magnesium ammonium phosphate (struvite)	10–20
Uric acid	5–10
Cystine	< 1

cystinuria, which is an autosomal defect in the transport of the amino acids cystine, ornithine, lysine and arginine in the kidney and intestine.

Rarely, drugs can crystallize in the urine and form stones (e.g. indinavir, triamterene, aciclovir).

Risk factors

The most important risk factors for kidney stones are the supersaturation of urine with calcium oxalate and/or uric acid, and the pH of the urine (Table 10.2); however, other underlying risk

TABLE 10.2

Risk factors for kidney stone formation

Risk factor	Example
Supersaturation of urine with solute	• Hypercalciuria • Hyperoxaluria
Inadequate inhibition of stone formation	• Hypocitraturia • Reduced urinary osteopontin
Anatomic abnormalities	• Pyelocalyceal diverticula • Pelviureteric junction obstruction • Horseshoe kidney
Diet	• High protein intake, excess sodium, low urine volume (especially in stone-belt area in Southeastern USA and Middle East)
Urinary pH	• Urinary tract infection caused by urease-splitting organism promotes alkaline urine and struvite stone formation • Acid urine favors formation of uric acid and cystine stones
Medication	• Acetazolamide increases urine pH and calcium excretion • Triamterene crystallizes in urine and forms a nidus for stone formation • Vitamin C • Calcium and vitamin D • Theophylline

factors are incompletely understood. Reduced levels or absence
of urinary inhibitors of stone formation, such as citrate, also favor
stone formation. Urinary infection with a urease-splitting organism
is a key factor in struvite stone formation.

Pathophysiology

Calcium stone disease. The most common stones are calcium
oxalate stones rather than pure calcium phosphate. The major cause
of calcium stone formation is excessive urinary excretion of calcium
(hypercalciuria). This may occur with or without hypercalcemia.
(The most common cause of hypercalcemia is primary
hyperparathyroidism.) Hypercalciuria without hypercalcemia is
observed in 60% of patients with calcium stones. The primary
abnormality appears to be impairment in renal tubular resorption
of calcium, but it also reflects increased absorption of dietary
calcium and excessive bone resorption. Other less common etiologies
include hyperuricosuria, which occurs in about 10% of patients,
hyperoxaluria, hypocitraturia and medullary sponge kidney.

Non-calcareous stone disease. The most common type of
non-calcareous stones are struvite stones, which are also termed
'infection' stones, because they are usually associated with
urinary tract infection by a urea-splitting organism. Bacterial
urease degrades urea into ammonia (and subsequently ammonium),
resulting in alkaline urine, which favors the formation of
triphosphate ions and reduces the solubility of struvite. Uric acid
stone formation is also critically dependent on the urinary pH.
A urinary pH lower than the dissociation constant for uric acid
(pH 5.5) and/or the presence of hyperuricosuria play major roles
in uric acid stone formation. Chronic diarrheal syndromes, such
as ulcerative colitis and Crohn's disease, and jejunoileal bypass
surgery are associated with reduced urinary pH and thus a
greater propensity for uric acid stone formation. Hyperuricosuria
is most frequently observed in states of purine overproduction,
such as myeloproliferative states and glycogen storage

diseases.

Clinical features

The clinical presentation varies depending on the location, size and number of stones. The most common presentation is renal colic, which is the sudden onset of severe pain caused by the presence of an obstructing renal or ureteral stone. Renal colic is typically spasmodic, lasts several minutes, is localized to the flank and radiates down to the groin, accompanied by nausea and vomiting. It often occurs in the middle of the night or early morning while the patient is sedentary, and its severity has been described as akin to or worse than childbirth. On the other hand, larger stones may present with painless obstruction or back pain. Stones that reach the ureterovesical junction often present with renal colic accompanied by urgency and frequency. Stones located in the renal calyces may be completely asymptomatic. Patients with renal colic are often writhing in excruciating pain and restless. The presence of fever usually heralds an accompanying urinary tract infection. Otherwise, the physical examination may be completely unremarkable.

Diagnosis

Laboratory evaluation should include a complete blood count, blood chemistry including measurement of BUN (serum urea) and creatinine, and urinalysis (Table 10.3). The presence of a urinary tract infection, particularly with pyelonephritis, will be associated with a leukocytosis. An elevated BUN and creatinine would suggest dehydration and/or the presence of an obstructing stone in a patient with a single kidney, or bilateral obstructing stones. Hematuria and pyuria are usually present. Assessment of urine pH is critical, because acid urine with a radiolucent stone suggests a uric acid stone, while an alkaline urine (pH > 8.0) suggests infection with a urease-splitting organism (e.g. *Proteus, Pseudomonas, Klebsiella*). Imaging should include a radiograph of the kidney, ureters and bladder, and an ultrasound or a non-contrast computerized tomography (CT) scan (Figure 10.1).

Management

Initially, management is directed towards optimal pain control, hydration, and urologic consultation for potential removal of an

TABLE 10.3

Diagnosis of kidney stones

Identify the number, size and location of stones

- Radiopaque stones can be seen on a plain abdominal radiograph of the kidneys, ureters and bladder

- Radiolucent stones can be detected by ultrasound, computerized tomography or intravenous pyelography

- Imaging will also detect evidence of renal outflow obstruction

Analysis of the chemical composition of the stone

- Strain urine (use a coffee filter paper)

- Send stone to a specialist laboratory for stone analysis

Metabolic investigations

- Urinalysis, urine pH and urine culture

- Blood chemistry, including blood urea nitrogen (serum urea), creatinine, calcium, electrolytes, bicarbonate and complete blood count

- 24-hour urine collection for volume, pH, calcium, phosphorus, sodium, uric acid, oxalate, citrate, cystine and creatinine (collect at least two specimens to account for variability)

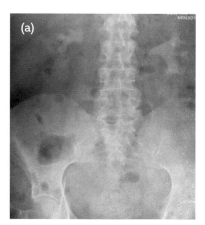 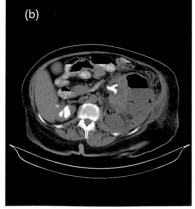

Figure 10.1 (a) Plain abdominal radiograph showing bilateral staghorn calculi; (b) CT scan of bilateral staghorn calculi and a secondary left renal abscess.

obstructing stone, and subsequently to the underlying predisposing factors and prevention of further episodes. Medical management of a non-obstructing stone requires increasing fluid intake to generate a urine output of more than 2 liters/day, dietary modification and treatment targeted at changing urinary pH (Tables 10.4 and 10.5). Low-calcium diets are to be avoided.

TABLE 10.4

Dietary modifications in the long-term management of kidney stones

High fluid intake
At least 10 glasses/day

Sodium restriction
Avoid salty foods, adding salt to meals and prepared meals

Oxalate restriction
Avoid nuts, spinach, chocolate, tea and vitamin C

Purine reduction
Reduce meat protein intake especially

High citrate intake
Increase intake of citrus fruits

TABLE 10.5

Management of kidney stone disease

Abnormality	Management
Calcium oxalate	
Hyperoxaluria	• Reduce oxalate intake (rhubarb, spinach, beetroot, chocolate, peanuts, strawberries, tea, wheat bran) • If ileal disease present, give oral calcium supplement and cholestyramine
Hyperuricosuria	• Allopurinol, 100–600 mg/day • Reduce purine intake (proteins) • Alkalinize urine to pH > 6.5 with sodium bicarbonate, 60–100 mmol/day

CONTINUED

TABLE 10.5 (CONTINUED)

Management of kidney stone disease

Abnormality	Management
Calcium oxalate	
Hypercalciuria	• Identify secondary causes and treat • Thiazide diuretic (e.g. hydrochlorthiazide, 50–100 mg/day in split doses, or chlorthalidone) stimulates calcium reabsorption • Cellulose sodium phosphate (calcibind) • Neutral potassium phosphate, 1500 mg in divided doses, may reduce hypercalciuria • Low-calcium diets are not useful; can demineralize skeleton, increase stone formation and increase oxalate absorption • Low-salt diet (< 2 g/day) reduces calcium excretion (and uric acid and oxalate)
Low urinary citrate	• Potassium citrate, 10–20 mmol three times daily with meals • Drinking a mixture of water, sugar and lemon juice increases urinary citrate and volume
Calcium phosphate	
Hypercalciuria	• As above • Treat underlying disorder (e.g. hyper-parathyroidism, renal tubular acidosis) • Stop acetazolamide • Potassium bicarbonate or citrate
Magnesium ammonium phosphate (struvite)	
Infection	• Remove all stone material followed by prolonged antibiotics to ensure urine sterility • If stones remain, prolong suppressive antibiotics • Urease inhibitor (acetohydroxamine) as adjunctive therapy

CONTINUED

TABLE 10.5 (CONTINUED)

Management of kidney stone disease

Abnormality	Management
Uric acid	
Hyperuricemia	• Increase hydration (urine output > 2 L/day) • Alkalinize urine with potassium citrate • Reduce meat intake • Allopurinol, 100–600 mg/day • Avoid uricosuric agents
Cystine	
Cystinuria	• Increase hydration (urine output > 2 L/day) • Reduce methionine-rich protein in diet • Raise urine pH to > 6.5 with sodium bicarbonate • Sulfahydryl-containing agent, such as penicillamine, 1–2 g/day, or tiopronin, 800 mg/day, but side effects common

Surgical management depends on the size, location and number of stones (Tables 10.6 and 10.7). Obstruction may require percutaneous nephrostomy. Surgical options include extracorporeal shock-wave lithotripsy (ESWL) and stone removal (percutaneous or transurethral). Rules of thumb are that cystine and calcium oxalate monohydrate stones are generally poorly broken up by ESWL, while calcium oxalate, struvite and uric acid stones are usually amenable to ESWL, as well as to removal by either the percutaneous or transurethral route, depending on the size and location of the stones.

TABLE 10.6

Indications for urologic consultation

• Stones > 5 mm in diameter

• Stones impacted for > 24 hours

• Evidence of significant obstruction

• Evidence of infection

TABLE 10.7

Surgical management of kidney stones

Location and size of stone	Management
Kidney	
< 0.5 cm, asymptomatic	Observe
0.5–2 cm	Consider ESWL
> 2 cm or lower pole and > 1 cm	Percutaneous approach or ESWL
Ureter	
< 0.5 cm	Conservative management – may pass spontaneously
> 0.5 cm or not progressing	Proximal – push back and then ESWL (or PCNL) Distal – ESWL or ureteroscopic removal

ESWL, extracorporeal shock-wave lithotripsy; PCNL, percutaneous nephrolithotomy.

Key points – kidney stones

- Kidney stones are common and are most often associated with hypercalciuria.
- Stones can be asymptomatic or cause a variety of clinical problems.
- Stones may require surgical intervention, but recurrence after surgery is common.
- High fluid intake and a low-salt and low-oxalate diet are the mainstays of management.
- Low-calcium diets should be avoided.
- Thiazide diuretics and potassium citrate are used in some patients.

Key references

Borghi L, Meschi T, Schianchi T et al. Medical treatment of nephrolithiasis. *Endocrinol Metab Clin North Am* 2002;31:1051–64.

Delvecchio FC, Preminger GM. Medical management of stone disease. *Curr Opin Urol* 2003; 13:229–33.

Urinary tract obstruction

Urinary tract obstruction or obstructive uropathy is defined as complete or partial obstruction of the flow of urine at any level of the urinary tract from the kidneys to the urethral meatus. Urinary tract obstruction is a relatively common cause of community-acquired ARF (10% of cases) with an incidence of 23 cases/million population. Urinary tract obstruction has a bimodal age distribution, and is common in children and the elderly (> 60 years of age). In children, congenital abnormalities of the urinary tract are particularly common, and include pelviureteric junction obstruction and vesicoureteric junction obstruction, such as an ectopic ureter, ureterocele or posterior urethral valves. In adults, the commonest causes are benign prostatic hyperplasia (BPH) in men and pelvic malignancies in women.

Causes. Urinary tract obstruction can be classified according to cause (congenital versus acquired), duration (acute versus chronic), degree (partial versus complete) and location (upper versus lower urinary tract). Major causes are summarized in Table 11.1. The most common mechanical cause is BPH. Common causes of functional bladder outlet obstruction include neurogenic bladders, detrusor sphincter dyssynergia and iatrogenic medical intervention, such as the use of anticholinergic drugs.

Pathophysiology. Three main points of physiological narrowing of the urinary tract present a high risk for obstruction: the pelviureteric junction, the crossing of the ureter over the common iliac vessels at the pelvic brim and the vesicoureteric junction. The functional effects of urinary tract obstruction are influenced by the level, severity and duration of obstruction. Short-term complete infravesical obstruction is invariably associated with ARF together with an enlarged bladder, hydroureter and hydronephrosis. These abnormalities are reversible and rarely associated with long-term sequelae if diagnosed and treated early.

TABLE 11.1

Causes of urinary tract obstruction

Intrinsic

Intraluminal causes

- Intratubular deposition of crystals (uric acid, sulfates)
- Stones
- Papillary tissue
- Blood clots

Intramural functional causes

- Ureter (ureteropelvic or ureterovesical dysfunction)
- Bladder (neurogenic) – spinal cord defect or trauma, diabetes, multiple sclerosis, Parkinson's disease, cerebrovascular accidents, drugs
- Bladder neck dysfunction

Intramural anatomic causes

- Tumors
- Infection
- Granuloma
- Strictures

Extrinsic

Originating in the reproductive system

- Prostate – benign hyperplasia, cancer
- Uterus – pregnancy, tumors, prolapse, endometriosis
- Ovary – abscess, tumor, cysts

Originating in the vascular system

- Aneurysms (aorta, iliac vessels)
- Aberrant arteries (pelviureteric junction)
- Venous (ovarian veins, retrocaval ureter)

Originating in the gastrointestinal tract

- Crohn's disease
- Pancreatitis
- Appendicitis
- Tumors

Originating in the retroperitoneal space

- Inflammation
- Fibrosis
- Tumors
- Hematomas

Long-term complete infravesical obstruction may result in ARF or subacute renal failure coupled with structural changes that are often irreversible.

Obstruction to outflow from the bladder leads to hypertrophied muscle and marked trabeculation of the bladder wall, mucosal diverticula and, ultimately, detrusor muscle decompensation. Progressive back-pressure on the ureter and kidneys results in hydroureteronephrosis. Increased intrarenal pressure precipitates a reduction in renal blood flow, progressive ischemia, compression of the papillae, decreased GFR and loss of parenchyma secondary to loss of nephrons. Angiotensin II plays a pivotal role in this process, driving inflammatory and profibrotic changes. The result of this heightened cytokine activity is progressive irreversible renal fibrosis.

Clinical features. The level of obstruction and its duration governs the clinical presentation of urinary tract obstruction (Table 11.2). If the obstruction is complicated by UTI then symptoms associated with the infection are also usually present.

Since lower tract obstruction in men is commonly due to prostatic enlargement, a digital rectal examination is essential; in women, a thorough pelvic examination is necessary to detect pelvic malignancies.

Diagnosis. Urinary tract obstruction should be sought in any individual who presents with renal failure of unknown cause. The history and physical examination are often crucial. Sudden onset of complete anuria is highly suggestive of urinary tract obstruction, and ultrasound examination is the preferred diagnostic investigation.

The finding of hydronephrosis in association with back-pressure changes in the renal parenchyma is central to the diagnosis. However, hydronephrosis is not always caused by obstruction. For example, vesicoureteric reflux, papillary necrosis, brisk diuresis in nephrogenic diabetes insipidus and pregnancy may cause calyceal dilatation in the absence of obstruction. Hydronephrosis should be categorized as either obstructive or non-obstructive. With obstructive hydronephrosis, the degree of dilatation of the pelvicalyceal system maybe an insensitive indicator of the severity of obstruction. Some patients with acute

TABLE 11.2

Clinical presentation of urinary tract obstruction

Acute upper tract obstruction

- Flank pain
- Palpable enlarged kidney

Lower urinary tract obstruction

- Voiding difficulty
- Hesitancy
- Dribbling
- Inadequate bladder emptying

Chronic obstruction

- Symptoms and signs of chronic renal failure (nausea, anorexia, weight loss, pruritus)

Chronic lower tract obstruction

- Urinary urgency
- Urge incontinence
- Bladder enlargement

complete obstruction may initially have mild or no hydronephrosis, because of the brief duration of the obstruction, low urine production or external compression from a retroperitoneal process. Thus, a normal ultrasound examination does not exclude obstruction.

In acute obstruction, the renal cortex is intact, whereas chronic obstruction usually leads to marked thinning of the cortex. Failure to visualize the proximal ureter suggests obstruction at the pelviureteric junction, whereas a dilated ureter indicates an obstruction downstream, often at the level of the bladder. A large postvoid bladder indicates urinary retention, often as a result of prostatic enlargement, whereas an empty bladder with dilatation of the distal ureters suggests obstruction at the bladder inlet. Therefore, it is essential to examine the entire urinary tract when hydronephrosis is present.

Once a diagnosis of urinary obstruction has been made, further investigations are necessary to establish the underlying cause (Table 11.3, Figure 11.1).

Contrast medium for intravenous urography or CT may lead to renal dysfunction in patients with existing renal impairment and should be administered with caution. In most circumstances, after renal ultrasonography, a CT scan followed by either antegrade or retrograde pyelography is the best approach. Assessment of lower tract obstruction to distinguish functional from mechanical causes may include uroflowmetry (to measure the speed of urine flow), postvoid residual

TABLE 11.3

Investigation of urinary tract obstruction

Urine

- Urinalysis
- Urine culture
- Urine cytology

Blood

- Renal function (blood urea nitrogen [serum urea] and creatinine)
- Prostate-specific antigen
- Serum tumor markers (CA-125)

Imaging

- Postvoid residual urine
- Renal ultrasonography
- Pelvic transvaginal ultrasonography
- Prostate ultrasonography
- Intravenous excretory urography
- Urethrocystoscopy (also called cystourethroscopy)

Assessment of function

- Uroflowmetry
- Filling cystometry (also called cystometrography)

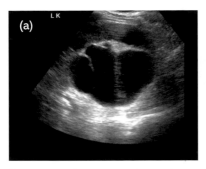 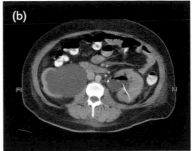

Figure 11.1 Imaging renal tract obstruction. (a) Ultrasound scan of an obstructed kidney; (b) CT scan showing bilateral obstruction, a chronically obstructed right kidney with thin cortex and gross hydronephrosis, and mild dilatation of the left kidney, with nephrostomy tube in situ.

urine measurement (to determine the amount of urine left in the bladder after urination) and filling cystometry (to determine the presence of uninhibited detrusor contractions).

Treatment. Most patients should be referred for urologic evaluation, because untreated obstruction may result in irreversible parenchymal renal injury. Immediate referral is particularly important if there is complete obstruction or if there are associated complications such as renal failure or infection (Table 11.4).

Obstruction coexisting with infection should be considered a urologic emergency and requires immediate relief with a Foley catheter, ureteral stent or percutaneous nephrostomy tube, and broad-spectrum antibiotics. In patients with partial obstruction, particularly in the

TABLE 11.4

Indications for expeditious intervention and/or hospitalization

- Complete obstruction
- Obstruction in a solitary kidney
- Associated sepsis
- Acute renal failure
- Uncontrolled colic and/or pain

setting of infection, initial management with analgesia and antibiotics is reasonable until a full evaluation can be completed. Colic secondary to urinary obstruction can be severe and is best managed with opioid analgesics, such as morphine sulfate, oxycodone and hydrocodone. NSAIDs or cyclo-oxygenase 2 inhibitors should be avoided if possible, because they may exacerbate or precipitate ARF. Antibiotic prophylaxis should be initiated to cover common urinary pathogens (e.g. trimethoprim, trimethoprim–sulfamethoxazole, cefalexin).

Surgical management may be temporary; for example, relieving the obstruction using a Foley catheter, ureteral stent or percutaneous nephrostomy tube. More definitive surgical intervention will depend on the cause, type and duration of obstruction.

Tumors of the urinary tract

Tumors of the urinary tract can involve the kidney, ureters, bladder, prostate or urethra. Only tumors of the kidney and prostate will be discussed here.

Tumors of the kidney

Benign tumors. The most common benign tumor is renal fibroma. It usually presents incidentally as a nodule less than 1 cm in diameter in the medulla or the papillae, and can usually be managed conservatively by observation. Cortical adenomas, though benign, are histologically indistinguishable from renal cell carcinoma and are usually resected surgically.

Malignant tumors. The most common malignant tumors are renal cell carcinoma and renal pelvic tumors in adults, and Wilm's tumor in children.

Renal cell carcinomas are relatively rare and account for only 1–3% of all visceral cancers. They occur most typically in males over 50 years of age. The clinical presentation is variable; tumors may be picked up incidentally or may present with hematuria, loin pain, as a mass or as a paraneoplastic syndrome (hypercalcemia, hypertension or polycythemia). Renal cell cancers often present late and have a relatively poor prognosis. In the absence of metastatic disease, 5-year survival is 70%, but with renal vein involvement or extension into perinephric fat, the 5-year survival is only 20%. Risk factors for renal cell carcinoma include smoking, obesity, acetaminophen (paracetamol) use, gasoline exposure, kidney stones and von Hippel–Lindau disease (approximately 30–50% of all patients). Treatment usually comprises radical nephrectomy.

Carcinoma of the renal pelvis is a transitional cell carcinoma arising from the urothelium. These tumors present early with hematuria or obstruction, and are often associated with similar tumors in the ureters and bladder. Risk factors include a history of analgesic abuse and exposure to aniline dye.

Wilm's tumors are the commonest intra-abdominal tumor in children under 10 years of age. Peak incidence occurs between the age of 1 and 4 years. The tumors may contain fibrous tissue, bone and fat. The child may present with an abdominal mass and pain, hematuria, hypertension or intestinal obstruction. Wilm's tumor is aggressive and at the time of diagnosis may have already spread to the lungs. Treatment includes chemotherapy and radiotherapy, which have both greatly improved the prognosis.

Prostatic tumors

Benign tumors. BPH is the most usual benign tumor. It is common in men over 50 years of age; indeed, 75% men over the age of 70 years have BPH. A hormonal imbalance of declining androgen levels and thus a relative increase in estrogen level is thought to result in hyperplasia of estrogen-sensitive periurethral glands of the prostate, as well as stromal tissue including smooth muscle and fibrous tissue. Clinical features in patients with early BPH include delay in starting micturition (hesitancy), a poor or intermittent stream, postmicturition dribbling and hematuria. Later, because of compression of the prostatic urethra by hyperplastic nodules or infarction of prostatic nodules, acute retention may develop. This can be associated with severe pain. If the obstruction occurs gradually, chronic retention ensues. This may be relatively painless, but is often associated with a history of increased frequency and overflow incontinence. The bladder is often palpable to the umbilicus.

Key points – urinary tract obstruction and tumors

- Urinary tract obstruction is common and can lead to irreversible renal failure if not recognized.
- An infected obstructed urinary system is a urological emergency.
- Renal cell carcinoma often presents late, while transitional cell carcinoma of the renal pelvis causes obstruction and presents early.
- Malignant prostate tumors are common, and are treated by antiandrogen therapy initially. The place of surgery remains controversial.

Chronic bladder outflow obstruction is associated with secondary changes in the bladder, including hypertrophy and trabeculation with development of diverticula that may protrude between bands of muscle, hydronephrosis and hydroureter. Management comprises temporary relief of acute obstruction by Foley catheterization, treatment of any associated infection with appropriate antibiotics and medical management with drugs aimed at reversing the hyperplasia (e.g. α-adrenergic blockers and antiandrogens). Nevertheless, a definitive surgical procedure is often necessary; options include transurethral prostatectomy or open prostatectomy.

Malignant tumors. The most usual malignant tumor is prostatic adenocarcinoma. Among men over 50 years of age, prostatic adenocarcinoma is one of the commonest forms of malignant disease; it is the fifth most frequent cause of malignant death in males in the UK. Risk factors include the presence of BPH, because both conditions often coexist, though there is little evidence to suggest that BPH is premalignant.

There are two types of prostatic carcinoma. Clinical or active adenocarcinoma is very well differentiated. It arises in the periphery of the posterior lobe (not usually periurethral) and disrupts the architecture of the gland by obliterating the median groove of the prostate. It metastasizes to bone, but may also spread directly through the capsule to the urethra, bladder and the seminal vesicle. Spread may also occur via the lymphatics to sacral, iliac or pre-aortic nodes or hematogenously to bone. The second type of prostatic adenocarcinoma is a latent or incidental carcinoma. It is often found as a microscopic focus either incidentally or at postmortem. Latent prostatic adenocarcinoma has no clinical symptoms. It has a very high incidence in old age; it is seen in 30% of those over 50 years of age and 80% of those over 75 years of age. It is usually 'dormant', does not metastasize and has an uncertain natural history. Treatment is seldom necessary.

Detection of prostatic adenocarcinoma has been helped by the widespread availability of assays for prostate-specific antigen. However, its use as a screening tool remains controversial. Digital rectal examination and ultrasound of the prostate continue to be important. Treatment strategies include reduction of androgen levels by means of estrogens, orchiectomy or cyproterone (a progestogen antiandrogen competitive antagonist). Radiotherapy provides effective palliation for bone metastases.

Key references

Hernandez J, Thompson IM. Prostate-specific antigen: a review of the validation of the most commonly used cancer biomarker. *Cancer* 2004;101:894–904.

Naderi N, Mochtar CA, de la Rosette JJ. Real life practice in the management of benign prostatic hyperplasia. *Curr Opin Urol* 2004; 14:41–4.

Renal disease can affect the outcome of pregnancy, pregnancy can affect the progression of preexisting renal disease and pregnancy can itself cause renal impairment.

Renal function in pregnancy

During a normal pregnancy in a woman with normal kidneys, renal plasma flow and glomerular filtration both increase (by $\geq 50\%$), leading to a reduction in the mean serum creatinine during the first and second trimesters from 73 µmol/L (0.8 mg/dL) to 51 µmol/L (0.5 mg/dL). If serum creatinine does not fall during pregnancy, this can indicate significant renal functional impairment. Glycosuria is common and does not usually indicate diabetes or even impaired glucose tolerance. Urinary protein excretion increases during pregnancy, but never to more than 300 mg/day, and therefore overt proteinuria is not physiological. Women are at increased risk of UTI, because of renal tract dilatation leading to urinary stasis, and this should be treated promptly according to bacterial sensitivity.

Pregnancy in patients with preexisting renal disease

Women with only mild renal impairment from any cause will usually have a successful pregnancy outcome, and will seldom incur any additional renal damage as a result of the pregnancy. Some women, however, will have complications during the pregnancy itself, especially hypertension. Women with more severe renal impairment are more likely to suffer hypertension, preeclampsia or premature labor, and to have a small baby, miscarriage or irreversible decline in renal function in the long term (Table 12.1).

Pregnancy is extremely uncommon in women with ESRF on dialysis, for a variety of reasons; most such women are infertile. Fertility often returns rapidly after a successful renal transplant. If women on dialysis do become pregnant, the outcome is usually poor with a very high risk

TABLE 12.1

Pregnancy outcomes for women with preexisting renal disease

Creatinine level	Problems during pregnancy	Successful obstetric outcome	Long-term problems
< 125 µmol/L (1.4 mg/dL)	26%	96%	< 3%
125–250 µmol/L (1.4–2.8 mg/dL)	47%	89%	25%
> 250 µmol/L (2.8 mg/dL)	88%	46%	53%

of miscarriage, severe hypertension, small babies and prematurity. Only 47% of women have a successful obstetric outcome.

Medications, especially antihypertensive agents, must be reviewed in women with renal disease who wish to get pregnant, and additional aspirin, anticoagulation or antibiotic prophylaxis may be required (Table 12.2).

Pregnancy-induced renal disease

Pregnancy itself can cause acute renal failure (Table 12.3), and renal disease can present for the first time during pregnancy. Women should be investigated as normal; renal biopsy, if indicated, is safe.

Hypertension in pregnancy

Hypertension during pregnancy is defined as any rise in systolic blood pressure of more than 30 mmHg or a rise in diastolic blood pressure of more than 15 mmHg above baseline, or the use of antihypertensive agents. It is classified according to its presentation (Table 12.4). Chronic hypertension is more common in multiparous women, and is present at the first antenatal visit. On the other hand, preeclampsia is more common in primigravidas (it occurs in 10% of first pregnancies), and represents an important cause of maternal and perinatal mortality. It usually presents only after 20 weeks of gestation, with or without

TABLE 12.2

Problems related to specific kidney diseases in pregnancy

Reflux nephropathy
- Prophylactic antibiotics
- Potential for inheritance

Systemic lupus erythematosus
- High risk of spontaneous abortion
- May need immunosuppression
- Problems for fetus (e.g. neonatal lupus, heart block)

Diabetic nephropathy
- Worse hypertension
- Increased risk of preeclampsia
- Accelerated decline in renal function

Kidney transplant recipient
- Increased risk of miscarriage in first trimester
- Risk from some immunosuppressants (e.g. mycophenolate mofetil)
- Increased hypertension
- Premature delivery

proteinuria and a raised serum urate. Preeclampsia may progress to full-blown eclampsia, which is characterized by seizures and also associated with acute renal failure. Management of eclampsia comprises immediate delivery, and magnesium sulfate, anticonvulsant and antihypertensive therapy.

Methyldopa, labetalol, hydralazine and nifedipine are all safe drugs for treating hypertension in pregnancy, but diuretics should be avoided. ACE inhibitors are contraindicated from the second trimester, but may be important in controlling the progression of CKD. Women may therefore continue to take these as they plan a pregnancy but must stop when pregnant.

TABLE 12.3

Causes of acute renal failure in pregnancy

- Hemorrhage
- Hyperemesis
- Abruption
- Preeclampsia
- Hemolytic uremic syndrome
- Pyelonephritis
- Acute fatty liver of pregnancy
- Sepsis (including septic abortion)
- Acute hydronephrosis
- Trauma (e.g. damage to ureter during surgery)

TABLE 12.4

Classification of hypertension during pregnancy

Classification	Definition
Chronic hypertension	Hypertension present before pregnancy or diagnosed before the 20th week of gestation that persists for > 6 weeks postpartum
Pregnancy-induced hypertension	Hypertension detected for the first time after the 20th week of gestation
Preeclampsia	Hypertension detected for the first time after the 20th week of gestation associated with proteinuria
Eclampsia	Preeclampsia with seizures that cannot be attributed to other causes

Key points – pregnancy

- Failure of creatinine to fall during pregnancy may indicate significant renal disease.
- Pregnant women with significant renal impairment are likely to have hypertension, preeclampsia and premature labor.
- Pregnancy can induce a number of renal diseases.
- Medications require careful review in pregnant women with renal disease.

Key references

Baylis C. Impact of pregnancy on underlying renal disease. *Adv Ren Replace Ther* 2003;10:31–9.

Higgins JR, de Swiet M. Blood-pressure measurement and classification in pregnancy. *Lancet* 2001;357:131–5.

Sanders CL, Lucas MJ. Renal disease in pregnancy. *Obstet Gynecol Clin North Am* 2001;28:593–600.

13 Renal replacement therapy and renal transplantation

Three choices for renal replacement therapy are available for patients with ESRF:
- conservative care and symptom control
- dialysis (either peritoneal or hemodialysis)
- kidney transplant (from a living or cadaveric donor).

In general, all patients should be offered all suitable choices, and be fully counseled as to the advantages and disadvantages of each. In reality, however, not all options are available in all centers, and patient-related factors can be limiting.

Conservative care in ESRF

Dialysis may not improve quality of life in patients with extensive comorbidities. Indeed, there is some evidence that very elderly patients, with only limited comorbid illnesses, may not even have the length of their lives prolonged by dialysis. In these circumstances, many patients opt for symptom control without dialysis, using erythropoietin, vitamin D analogs, dietary control, antipruritics and antiemetics as necessary. Such patients often have significantly better quality of life, fewer hospital admissions (e.g. from dialysis-related complications), and are more likely to die finally at home rather than in hospital than patients receiving dialysis.

Conservative care does not represent an absence of renal support, but rather the active medical (non-technological) management of the complications of renal failure. It is clearly important that patients participate fully in these discussions wherever possible. A multidisciplinary team approach is crucial and should involve nurses, doctors, counselors and family members.

Dialysis

The term dialysis refers to the physical process of the diffusion of a molecule down its concentration gradient, from an area of high concentration to an area of lower concentration, through a semipermeable membrane.

Hemodialysis involves pumping blood from the body through an artificial kidney in which the blood is surrounded by a solution of electrolytes, called the dialysate, whose concentration can be varied precisely. Solutes present in the blood at high concentration (e.g. urea, potassium, creatinine) diffuse into the dialysate and are removed (Figure 13.1).

Changing the concentration of solutes in the dialysate can alter the electrolyte composition of the blood. Raising the dialysate calcium above the serum concentration, for example, can increase serum calcium in patients with hypocalcemia.

A separate biophysical process, ultrafiltration, is used to regulate the distribution of water between the blood and dialysate. The volume of water to be removed from the patient's blood can be controlled by altering the pressures on either side of the membrane separating the blood from the dialysate.

The dialysis machine itself is simply the housing for the pumps controlling blood and dialysate flow, various safety devices (pressure

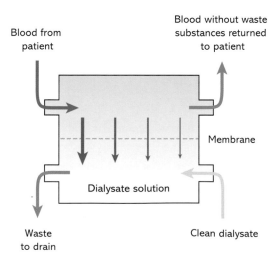

Figure 13.1 The principle of hemodialysis.

sensors, air detectors), a system for maintaining blood anticoagulation in the extracorporeal circuit (usually a heparin infusion), and a screen for graphically displaying the various parameters monitored. Different modalities of dialysis differ in the precise balance of ultrafiltration and dialysis, the speed of blood flow and the nature of the dialysate.

Patients need excellent vascular access, and access problems are a major cause of morbidity (Table 13.1). Access is obtained through either a fistula created between a peripheral artery and vein (usually radial or brachial), or a permanent plastic catheter inserted into an internal jugular or subclavian vein (Figure 13.2).

TABLE 13.1

Complications of hemodialysis

Access related

- Local infection
- Sepsis and bacteremia
- Endocarditis and osteomyelitis
- Fistula stenosis or thrombosis
- Superior vena cava, subclavian or internal jugular vein stenosis
- Fistula aneurysm formation

Complications during hemodialysis

- Hypotension
- Cardiac arrhythmias
- Nausea and vomiting
- Headache
- Cramps
- Fever
- Allergic reactions (e.g. to dialysers, tubing)
- Air embolism
- Heparin-induced thrombocytopenia
- Seizures
- Hemolysis

Hemodialysis can be carried out in a main hospital center, a satellite unit (often staffed only by nurses) or in the patient's home. Home hemodialysis offers patients the most autonomy, but requires a suitable house with a water supply, space (for the machine and supplies), a reasonably technically competent patient and a trained helper who will be present during each dialysis session. Patients dialysing at home often have the best quality of life. Dialysis is usually performed three times each week for about 4 hours. Some patients opt for daily hemodialysis

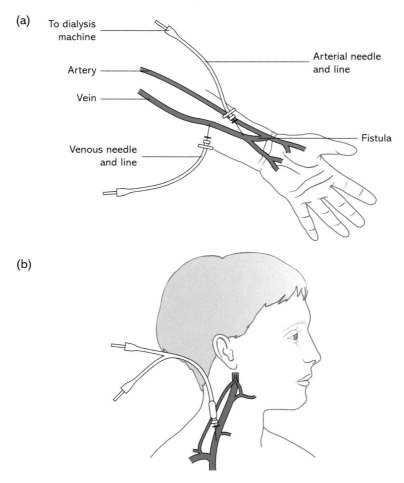

Figure 13.2 (a) Forearm arteriovenous fistula for hemodialysis; (b) internal jugular catheter for hemodialysis.

(usually 6 days/week), which provides the best control of fluid balance and biochemistry, but is intensive. It is difficult to determine the optimum amount of dialysis a patient requires, and various methods are in use.

Peritoneal dialysis uses the peritoneal cavity as a reservoir into which a dialysate can be infused, and the blood flowing through peritoneal capillaries as the blood source. Dialysis and ultrafiltration occur across these capillaries. Ultrafiltration is controlled by altering the osmolality of the dialysate solution and thus drawing water out of the patient's blood. This can be achieved with glucose or other large molecular weight solutes in the dialysate. The glucose load can cause problems of its own, such as poor diabetic control and weight gain.

A catheter is inserted into the patient's peritoneum under local or general anesthetic, which remains in place permanently and through which dialysate is infused. The waste solutes are removed by exchanging the peritoneal fluid for a fresh solution (Figure 13.3). As long as patients have reasonable manual dexterity, they can be trained to perform continuous ambulatory peritoneal dialysis (CAPD), typically four exchanges spaced throughout the day with each one taking about 20 minutes, or to use a machine (automated peritoneal dialysis, APD) to do a number of exchanges overnight while they sleep, and then perform only one or two daytime exchanges.

Peritoneal dialysis is carried out by the patient at home, at work or while on holiday. It therefore allows the patient a high degree of independence and control over their own illness. However, patients must not be allowed to become isolated, and still need considerable support.

Intra-abdominal adhesions and abdominal wall stoma are absolute contraindications for peritoneal dialysis, and obesity, intestinal disease, respiratory disease and hernias are relative contraindications. The complications of peritoneal dialysis are listed in Table 13.2.

When to start dialysis

The question of when to start dialysis remains controversial. In general, patients should begin dialysis when their GFR reaches 10 mL/minute,

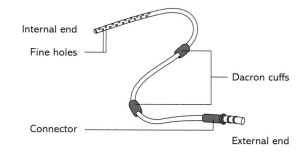

Internal end

Fine holes

Dacron cuffs

Connector

External end

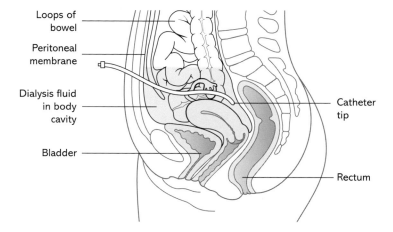

Loops of bowel

Peritoneal membrane

Dialysis fluid in body cavity

Bladder

Catheter tip

Rectum

Figure 13.3 Design and position of a peritoneal dialysis catheter.

TABLE 13.2

Complications of peritoneal dialysis

- Peritonitis
- Catheter infection
- Catheter blockage, kinking, leaks or slow drainage
- Constipation
- Fluid retention
- Hyperglycemia

- Weight gain
- Hernias (incisional, inguinal, umbilical)
- Back pain
- Malnutrition
- Sclerosing peritonitis (rare)

or 15 mL/minute if they are diabetic. There is no good evidence that starting dialysis earlier is of any benefit to patients. If dialysis is delayed for too long, however, patients can become very malnourished. Nevertheless, there are excellent data suggesting that earlier referral for nephrological care before renal replacement therapy is required can significantly delay the need for dialysis, and reduce early morbidity and mortality.

Transplantation

A kidney transplant provides the best long-term outcome for patients with ESRF. A transplant can come from a cadaveric donor, from a living relative or from an unrelated living donor (often called emotionally related). The sale of organs for transplantation is prohibited in almost all countries, but nevertheless continues, mostly because of the severe shortage of organs. All patients with ESRF should be considered for a transplant. Age itself is not a major determinant of outcome, though the presence of comorbid disease adversely affects survival (Table 13.3).

Patients should be aware of the risks and benefits of transplantation (Table 13.4), and require screening for occult cardiovascular disease before surgery. Over 90% of transplants should be working 1 year after surgery. A cadaveric transplant should have a mean survival of 15 years and a living transplant about 18–20 years.

TABLE 13.3

Contraindications for transplantation

- Cancer
- Active infection
- Uncontrolled ischemic heart disease
- Aquired immunodeficiency disease with opportunistic infections
- Active viral hepatitis
- Extensive peripheral vascular disease
- Mental incapacity

TABLE 13.4

Risks and benefits of kidney transplantation

Risks

- Immediate operative complications (local infection, pain, pneumonia, deep-vein thrombosis)
- Immediate graft failure
- Arterial or venous thrombosis in the transplant
- Infections (viral, bacterial, fungal)
- Cancer (skin, lymphoma)
- Side effects of immunosuppressive drugs (common)
- Death at time of surgery (rare)

Benefits

- Cessation of dialysis
- Improved quality of life
- Reversal of anemia
- Reversal of renal bone disease
- Normalization of diet
- Relaxation of fluid restriction

Patients do not generally have their native kidneys removed, and the transplanted kidney is placed extraperitoneally in the iliac fossa. Patients can usually expect to stay in hospital for 1–3 weeks, and require frequent follow-up after discharge (two or three times each week initially). Patients will be treated with a cocktail of immunosuppressant drugs, which may include ciclosporin, azathioprine, mycophenolate mofetil, tacrolimus, sirolimus or prednisolone. These drugs must be taken for life and require careful monitoring (Table 13.5).

Common complications. Routine postoperative problems, such as deep-vein thrombosis, pulmonary embolism and pneumonia, can occur. Specific problems include opportunistic infections (viral, fungal,

TABLE 13.5

Side effects of immunosuppressant drugs

All drugs

- Increased risk of infections
- Increased risk of malignancy (especially skin cancer and lymphoma)

Prednisolone

- Diabetes
- Osteoporosis
- Weight gain
- Hypertension
- Poor wound healing

Ciclosporin

- Hyperkalemia
- Tremor
- Neuropathy
- Hirsutism
- Nephrotoxicity
- Hypertension
- Dyslipidemia
- Gingival hypertrophy

Mycophenolate mofetil

- Diarrhea
- Constipation
- Nausea
- Leukopenia, anemia, thrombocytopenia

Azathioprine

- Hypersensitivity reactions
- Bone marrow suppression
- Hepatotoxicity
- Hair loss
- Colitis and pancreatitis

Tacrolimus

- Gastrointestinal disturbance
- Nephrotoxicity
- Hypertension
- Tremor
- Hirsutism
- Dyslipidemia
- Diabetes

Sirolimus

- Hyperlipidemia
- Thrombocytopenia
- Leukopenia
- Mouth ulcers
- Poor wound healing

TABLE 13.6

Complications of renal transplantation

Complication	Prevention	Management
Early (days)		
Immediate surgical complications	Heparin, wound care, physiotherapy	As normal
Urinary infection		Early detection and treatment
1–4 weeks		
Viral infections (especially herpes simplex virus)	Aciclovir prophylaxis	Aciclovir
Graft rejection	Immunosuppression drug monitoring	Corticosteroids, adjust immunosuppression
Acute tubular necrosis	Blood pressure control, fluid balance	Treat cause
Ciclosporin nephrotoxicity	Immunosuppression drug monitoring	Immunosuppression drug monitoring
Urinary obstruction	Ureteric stent insertion	Early detection, cystoscopy, stent
Later		
Opportunistic infections	Avoid over-immunosuppression	Treat infection aggressively
Rejection	Immunosuppression drug monitoring	Corticosteroids, adjust immunosuppression
Ciclosporin nephrotoxicity	Immunosuppression drug monitoring	Immunosuppression drug monitoring
Bone marrow suppression	Avoid overimmuno-suppression, monitor with complete blood count	Reduce drug dose, may need bone marrow examination
Cytomegalovirus infection	Ganciclovir prophylaxis	Ganciclovir
Lymphoma	Avoid over-immunosuppression	Reduce drug doses; may need chemotherapy

---

Key points – renal replacement therapy and renal transplantation

- Not all patients with end-stage renal failure need or want dialysis, and some may be managed conservatively.
- Most patients will require several modalities of renal replacement therapy in their lifetime.
- Hemodialysis requires excellent vascular access; problems with access cause significant morbidity.
- Peritoneal dialysis is an excellent modality for many patients, especially early in their end-stage renal disease.
- Transplantation offers the best long-term outcomes, but at the expense of long-term side effects from immunosuppression, including cancers and infections.

---

bacterial), malignancies (especially skin cancers), drug toxicity, recurrence of the original disease in the transplant, cardiovascular disease, hypertension, dyslipidemia and graft failure (Table 13.6). Patients should be followed up for life and undergo annual screening for cancers, drug toxicity and cardiovascular disease in addition to routine clinic visits. Most patients with a transplant will die from cardiovascular disease, which should, therefore, be aggressively managed.

Key references

Levy JB, Morgan J, Brown EA. *Oxford Handbook of Dialysis.* 2nd edn. Oxford: OUP, 2004.

Magee CC, Pascual M. Update in renal transplantation. *Arch Intern Med* 2004;164:1373–88.

Pierratos A. New approaches to hemodialysis. *Annu Rev Med* 2004;55:179–89.

Teitelbaum I, Burkart J. Peritoneal dialysis. *Am J Kidney Dis* 2003;42: 1082–96.

UK Renal Registry www.renalreg.com

Useful addresses

American Association of
Kidney Patients
3505 E Frontage Rd, Suite 315
Tampa, FL 33607-1796
Tel: +1 813 636 8100/
1 800 749 2257
Fax: +1 813 636 8122
www.aakp.org

American Society of Nephrology
1725 I Street, NW, Suite 510
Washington, DC 20006
Te: + 1 202 659 0599
Fax: +1 202 659 0709
www.asn-online.org

International Society of Nephrology
Avenue des Gaulois 7
B-1040 Brussels
Belgium
Phone: + 32 (0)2 7431546
Fax: + 32 (0)2 7431550
www.isn-online.org

British Renal Society
26 Oriental Road
Woking, Surrey GU22 7AW
www.britishrenal.org

National Kidney Federation (UK)
6 Stanley Street
Worksop S81 7HX
Tel: +44 (0)1909 487795
Fax: +44 (0)1909 481723
Helpline 0845 601 02 09
nkf@kidney.org.uk
www.kidney.org.uk

National Kidney Foundation (USA)
30 East 33rd St
New York, NY 10016
Tel: +1 212 889 2210/
1 800 622 9010
Fax: +1 212 689 9261
www.kidney.org

Renal Association (UK)
Unit 2, Triangle House
Broomhill Road
London SW18 4HX
Tel: +44 (0)870 833 2413
Fax: +44 (0)870 833 2434
www.renal.org
renal@trianglethree.com

Kidney Patient Guide
www.kidneypatientguide.org.uk

UK Renal Registry
www.renalreg.com

Nephron Information Center
nephron.com

UK Transplant
www.uktransplant.org.uk

Kidney Directions
www.kidneydirections.com

The Kidney Alliance (UK)
www.kidneyalliance.org.uk

Index

abnormalities 7, 25, 27, 34, 74
aciclovir 142
acid–base disorders 17, 29–31, 32
assessment of status 29
control 38
acidosis 24, 25, 26, 37, 38, 46, 53, 114
see also metabolic
acute cystitis
men 104, 107
women 101–3
acute kidney disease 14
acute renal failure (ARF) 4, 5, 15, 25, 33–9, 64, 123
causes 34, 118, 120, 124
in pregnancy 131
management 36–8
outcome 39
treatments 38–9
acute tubular necrosis (ATN) 4, 15, 33, 34, 35, 36, 89, 142
adenocarcinoma 126–7
adrenal failure 17
albumin 7, 12, 26, 27, 49, 55, 74, 78
albuminuria 66–8, 70, 72
aldosterone 17, 24, 25, 30, 31, 72
alkalosis 23
Alport's syndrome 10, 94, 96
see also hereditary nephritis
amiloride 25
aminoglycosides 34, 38
amoxicillin 102, 106
amyloidosis 8, 15, 89–90
analgesic abuse 10
anemia in CKD 46, 47–8, 51, 52, 56, 57
reversed by transplantation 140

aneurysms 14
angiography 13, 14, 35, 50, 63
angioplasty 14, 38, 64, 91
angiotension-converting enzyme (ACE) inhibitors 4, 25, 34, 45, 46, 47, 61, 62, 63, 70, 72, 87, 91, 94, 130
angiotension-receptor blockers (ARBs) 4, 47, 61, 62, 63, 70, 72, 73, 94
Anglo-Scandinavian Cardiac Outcome Trial (ASCOT) 60
anion gap 29, 30
antibiotics 101, 102, 103, 104, 105, 106, 107, 114, 123–4, 126, 129, 130
antidiuretic hormone (ADH) 4, 17
see also syndrome (SIADH)
anti-DNA antibodies 13, 36, 83
Antihypertensive and Lipid–Lowering Treatment to Prevent Heart Attack Trial (ALLHAT) 61
antihypertensive therapy 60–1, 129, 130
key features 62
antineutrophil cytoplasm antibody (ANCA) 4, 36, 77, 78, 80, 85
see also cytoplasmic ANCA; perinuclear ANCA
arrhythmias 22, 23, 34, 50, 135
atherosclerosis 61, 90–1
automated peritoneal dialysis (APD) 137

autosomal-dominant polycystic kidney disease (APKD) 4, 92–4
clinical features 92, 93
diagnosis 92–3
treatment 94
azathioprine 84, 86, 140
side effects 141

β–blockers 50, 61, 62, 65
B-cell dyscrasias 13
bacteremia 98, 105, 107, 135
bacteriuria 98, 101, 104, 106–7
asymptomatic 105–6
Bartter's syndrome 23, 24
bedside urine analysis 5
benefits of kidney transplantation 140
benign prostatic hyperplasia (BPH) 4, 118, 119, 125, 126
bisphosphonates 28
bladder carcinoma 10, 19, 34
bladder disease 10
blood glucose measurement 13
blood pressure in CKD 44–7, 51, 52, 57, 58–9, 60
blood tests 13, 35, 36
blood urea nitrogen (BUN) 4, 12, 43, 111, 112, 122
bone marrow suppression 142
burns 18, 20, 22, 34

C-reactive protein 103, 105
calcium-channel blocker 61, 62

calcium metabolism disorders 26–9, 49
hypercalcemia 28–9
hypocalcemia 26–8
calcium stones 108, 110
management 113–14, 115
calculi 10, 34, 93, 101, 112
see also kidney stones
Candida/yeasts 99, 100, 104
captopril 14, 65
cardiovascular factors in CKD 46, 48, 50–2, 56, 57
carpal tunnel syndrome 48, 54
casts in urine 7, 9, 11, 15, 35, 64, 78, 100, 105
catecholamines 23
catheter-associated UTI 106–7
catheter blockage/infection 138
causes of UTI 99
cells in urine 7, 9
see also casts
central pontine myelinolysis 20
chemotherapy 89, 125
children 17, 19, 21, 74, 75, 79, 80, 86, 94
and UTI 100, 105
UT obstruction 118
cholesterol emboli 34, 36, 90
chronic airway disease 31
chronic kidney disease (CKD) 4, 5, 14, 25, 33–4, 41–57, 58, 63, 96, 130
causes 43
clinical features 42
complications 47–56, 57
diagnosis 43–4
epidemic of 57
epidemiology 41–2, 57
incidence 57
management 44–7

Churg–Strauss syndrome 84, 85
Chvostek's sign 27, 31
ciclosporin 25, 34, 79, 142
side effects 141
ciprofloxacin 102
cirrhosis 18
clinical complications of UTI 101
clinical features and management of glomerulonephritis 78–81
clinical features of APKD 92, 93
of CKD 42–3
of diabetic nephropathy 67
of hereditary nephritis 94, 95
clinical symptoms 7
see also diseases and disorders by name
coagulation disturbances 10
Cockcroft–Gault formula 12
coma 21, 29, 31, 64
complement levels 13
complications 5
see also diseases and disorders by name
complications of CKD 47–56, 96
anemia 47–8, 57
cardiovascular 50–2, 57
dialysis amyloid 54–5
fluid overload/diet 55
investigations 48–9
malnutrition 55, 56
renal bone disease 52–4, 57
sexual/psychological/social 55
complications of hemodialysis 135
of peritoneal dialysis 138
of renal transplantation 142

computerized tomography (CT) 4, 13, 14, 51, 92, 100, 111, 122
conservative care in ESRF 133, 143
continuous ambulatory peritoneal dialysis (CAPD) 137
contrast medium 34, 35, 122
coronary heart disease 17
corticosteroids 28, 39, 53, 79, 87, 142
cortisol deficiency 18
creatinine clearance 9, 11, 12
creatinine measurement 9, 11, 12, 15, 33, 43, 44, 111, 112, 122, 128, 129, 132
Crohn's disease 110, 119
cryoglobulinemia 85, 87–8, 89
Waldenström's 88
crystals in urine 7, 36
Cushing's syndrome 24
cyclophosphamide 39, 79, 80, 81, 85–6, 88
as toxin 10
cystine stones 108–9, 115
cystitis 98, 101–4, 105
acute 102–3, 104
recurrent 103–4
symptoms 103
cystoscopy 122, 142
cysts 14, 41, 92–4
bone cysts 54
cytology 11, 122
cytoplasmic antineutrophil cytoplasm antibody (cANCA) 4, 85

deafness in hereditary nephritis 94, 95, 96
depression 55, 56
diabetes 5, 8, 10, 15, 42, 43, 51, 52, 57, 60, 63, 78, 119, 141
insipidus 20, 22, 120

diabetes (cont'd)
mellitus 13, 58, 65
diabetic nephropathy
65–73, 83, 130
epidemiology 65
natural history 66–8
prevention and
treatment 69–73
screening 68–9
diafiltration see
hemodialysis
diagnosis of CKD 43–4
of UTI 100
dialysis 5, 26, 36, 37,
38, 41, 42, 44, 45, 47,
81, 96, 128, 133–9
cost 44
peritoneal dialysis
137–9
see also hemodialysis
dialysis amyloid 54–5
diarrhea 18, 20, 22, 23,
24, 30, 34, 141
diet 8, 12, 43, 46, 49,
54, 55, 57, 71, 73,
109, 113, 114, 115,
133
see also nutrition
dietary modifications for
kidney stones 113
digital rectal
examination (DRE)
120, 127
digoxin 22, 23, 25
diltiazem 46
dipstick tests 7–8, 9, 68,
78, 100, 103
diuretics 18, 21, 22, 23,
26, 28, 31, 34, 37, 46,
55, 62, 63, 116, 130
see also thiazide
dopamine 37, 39
Doppler
ultrasonography 14,
35, 63
drugs as cause 8, 10, 34

edema 42, 48, 55, 61,
91
elderly people 17, 61,
84–5, 90, 105–6
electrocardiogram (ECG)
4, 22, 25, 26, 27, 49

electrolyte disturbances
17–29, 32
calcium metabolism
26–9
potassium disorders
21–6
sodium and water
disorders 17–21
electron microscopy 75,
94
embolization 14
see also cholesterol
end-stage renal failure
(ESRF) 4, 5, 41, 44,
47, 52, 55, 74, 79, 94,
95, 96, 128
causes 43
hypertension in 58, 59,
60
malnutrition in 56
renal replacement
therapy 133–43
endocarditis 107, 135
epidemiology of CKD
42
of diabetic nephropathy
65–6
erythrocyte
sedimentation rate
(ESR) 4, 83
erythropoietin 46, 47,
48, 49, 50, 133
Escherichia coli 99, 103,
105, 106
euvolemic hypernatremia
20, 21
euvolemic hyponatremia
18
extracorporeal shock-
wave lithotripsy
(ESWL) 4, 115, 116
extrinsic causes of UT
obstruction 119

false-negative results 8
false-positive results 8
familial/hereditary
disease 43, 51
see also inherited
fluid balance 32, 37, 38,
55, 137
fluid retention 33, 38,
74, 138

fluoroquinolones 94,
106
see also quinolones
furosemide 14, 28, 39

gastrointestinal
hemorrhage 34, 38
gastrointestinal
symptoms of
hypercalcemia 28, 29
genetic analysis 93, 95–6
genetic counseling 96
glomerular basement
membrane (GBM) 81,
85, 94, 96
glomerular
disease/damage 7, 9,
10, 15, 34, 66, 78
glomerular filtration rate
(GFR) 4, 9, 11, 12, 15,
22, 25, 29, 120
in ARF 33
in CKD 41, 43–4, 45,
47, 50, 52
in glomerulonephritis
74, 78
in pregnancy 128
when to start dialysis
137, 139
glomerular hematuria 9
glomerular proteinuria 7
glomerulonephritis 8, 9,
10, 13, 15, 34, 35, 39,
42, 43, 74–82
see also
mesangiocapillary
glomerulonephritis
Goodpasture's syndrome
10, 36, 76, 77, 81
graft failure/rejection
140, 142, 143
Guillain–Barré syndrome
19

healthcare expenditure
on UTI 98
heart failure 17
heavy metals as toxins 8,
34, 35
hematuria 7, 9, 15, 34,
64, 74, 75, 78, 79, 80,
93, 94, 95, 96, 100,
103, 111, 124, 125

hematuria *(cont'd)*
  causes 10
  investigation
    algorithms 9, 11
hemodialysis 41, 47, 55,
  134–7, 143
  complications 135
hemoglobin 9, 35, 49
hemoglobinuria 8
hemolysis 9, 25, 26, 35,
  47, 55, 135
hemolytic uremic
  syndrome (HUS) 4, 34,
  39, 86–7, 131
Henoch–Schönlein
  purpura 10, 80, 85
hepatitis 79, 139
  vaccination 47
hepatorenal syndrome
  34
hereditary nephritis 10
  clinical features 94, 95
  diagnosis 95–6
  management 96
  see also Alport's
    syndrome
herpes simplex virus
  (HSV) 142
histological patterns in
  glomerulonephritis
  75–7
Hodgkin's disease 79
  non-Hodgkin's
    lymphoma 88
human
  immunodeficiency virus
  (HIV) 4, 49, 79
hydronephrosis 118,
  120–1, 123, 126, 131
hypercalcemia 28–9, 87,
  89, 110, 124
  causes 28
  clinical manifestations
    29
hypercalciuria 109, 110,
  114
hyperglycemia 69, 138
hypericosuria 110, 113
hyperkalemia 23, 25–4,
  38, 72, 141
  causes 25
  treatment 26
hypernatremia 20–1

hyperosmolality *see*
  hypernatremia
hyperoxaluria 109, 110,
  113
hyperparathyroidism 28,
  47, 51, 52, 53, 54, 56,
  110, 114
hyperphosphatemia 46,
  52, 54
hypertension 5, 42, 43,
  48, 50, 51, 52, 55, 57,
  58–65, 74, 75, 91, 93,
  94, 96, 124, 141, 143
  malignant 10, 34, 61
  pregnancy and 128,
    129–31, 132
hypertension and
  diabetic nephropathy
  69, 71–3
hypertensive emergencies
  64–5
hyperventilation 31
hypervolemic
  hypernatremia 20, 21
hypoaldosteronism *see*
  aldosterone
hypocalcemia 26–8, 52,
  53, 54
  causes 27
  treatment 27–8
hypokalemia 21–4, 62
  causes 22, 23, 24
  clinical features 21–2
  diagnosis 22, 23, 24
  treatment 23–4
hyponatremia 17–20
  clinical features 17
  diagnosis 17–18
  treatment 19–20
hypo-osmolality *see*
  hyponatremia
hypoparathyroidism 27,
  28
hypotension 34, 135
hypothyroidism 17, 18
hypovolemic
  hypernatremia 20, 21
hypervolemic
  hyponatremia 18

IgA nephropathy 80, 95
immunofluorescence 76,
  77, 85

immunoglobin (Ig) 4,
  35, 83
immunohistochemistry
  75
immunohistology 77, 95
immunological tests 13
immunosuppression/
  -compromise 80, 82,
  106, 107, 130, 142
  side effects 140, 141
  infection 9, 10, 34, 38,
    43, 55, 79, 80, 86, 88,
    93, 94, 114, 115, 119,
    123–4, 126, 135, 139,
    140, 141
inflammation of urinary
  tract 7, 8, 10, 119, 120
inherited kidney disease
  92–6
  autosomal-dominant
    polycystic (APKD)
    92–94, 96
  hereditary nephritis
    94–6
insulin/dextrose 26, 37
interstitial disease 10,
  15, 34, 36, 39, 89
intrinsic ARF 33, 34, 35
intrinsic causes of UT
  obstruction 119
iohexol clearance 12

Joint National
  Committee on the
  Prevention, Detection,
  Evaluation and
  Treatment of High
  Blood Pressure 58, 72

ketoacidosis 30
kidney stones 100,
  108–15, 119
  pathophysiology 110
  see also calculi
kidney tumors 124–5
  benign 124
  malignant 124–5
Klebsiella 99, 105, 111

left ventricular
  hypertrophy 42–3, 48,
  49, 50, 51, 52, 64
light microscopy 75

low-density lipoprotein
(LDL) 4, 68, 70
lymphoma 140, 142
lymphoproliferative
diseases 88

magnetic resonance
imaging (MRI) 14, 35
malignancy 9, 18, 27,
28, 141, 143
malnutrition 23, 46, 49,
51, 52, 55, 73
causes in ESRF 56
in dialysis patients 138,
139
management 5
management of CKD
44–7
management of kidney
stones 111–15
surgical 115–16, 117
management strategies in
diabetic nephropathy
71
medical costs 5
medullary sponge kidney
10
mesangiocapillary
glomerulonephritis
(MCGN) 4, 76, 79–80,
88
metabolic acidosis 24,
29, 30–1, 56
metabolic alkalosis 24,
31
microscopic polyangiitis
84, 85
mithramycin 28
modification of diet in
renal disease (MDRD)
4, 12
monoclonal
dysproteinemias 88–9
monoclonal
immunoglobulin
deposition disease 8
morbidity 5,17, 38, 47,
48, 55, 60, 98, 104,
135, 143
mortality 5, 17, 21, 39,
48, 50, 55, 60
multidisciplinary team
approach 133

mycophenolate mofetil
83, 130, 140
side effects 141
myeloma 7, 8, 13, 34,
35, 36, 78, 88–9
myoglobin 9, 35
myoglobinuria 8, 38

National Kidney
Foundation (USA) 41,
45, 144
natural history of
diabetic nephropathy
66–8
neoplastic disorders and
SIADH 19
nephrostomy 14
percutaneous 36
nephritic syndrome 9,
18, 74, 78, 79
nephrotoxins 34, 35, 37,
38, 94, 141
neurological disorders
and SIADH 19
neurological features of
hypercalcemia 28, 29
non-calcium phosphate
binders 54
non-steroidal anti-
inflammatory drugs
(NSAIDs) 4, 25, 34,
35, 38, 72, 124
nutrition 20, 37, 38, 55,
73
see also diet

obesity 51, 52, 57, 71,
125, 137
obstruction 14, 15, 34,
35, 36, 43, 99, 112,
115, 118–24
obstructive uropathy 89,
118, 142
ocular changes in
hereditary nephritis 94,
95, 96
oliguria 36–7, 39
opioid analgesics 124
opportunistic infections
140, 142
organisms in urine 7
osteitis fibrosa 53
osteodystrophy 52

osteomalacia 53, 54
osteopenia 53
osteoporosis 53, 141
overflow proteinuria 7,
8

Paget's disease 28
pancreatitis 27, 29, 119,
141
papillary necrosis 10
paralysis 22, 26
parathyroid hormone
(PTH) 4, 49, 52–3, 54
level 28
parenteral drugs 64–5
pelvic disease 10
penicillin 25, 105
perinuclear
antineutrophil
cytoplasm antibody
(pANCA) 4, 85
peritoneal dialysis 137,
138, 143
complications 138
contraindications 137
plasma exchange 39, 81,
86, 87, 88, 89
polycystic kidney disease
10, 106
adult 34
postrenal ARF 33, 34,
35–6
potassium disorders
21–6, 49
hyperkalemia 25–6
hypokalemia 21–4
prednisolone 39, 79, 80,
83, 84, 85, 88, 140
methyl- 81, 86
side effects 141
pregnancy 18, 106, 120
ectopic 105
hypertension in 65,
129–30
safe drugs for 130
renal disease and
128–32
UTI 106
pregnancy outcomes
128–9
abortion 130
miscarriage 128, 129,
130

pregnancy outcomes
(cont'd)
problems 128–9
long-term 128, 129
preeclampsia 128, 130,
131, 132
premature labor 128,
130, 132
success 128
pregnancy-induced renal
disease 129
preexisting renal disease
and pregnancy 128–9
outcomes 129
prerenal ARF 33, 34,
36
presentation of
glomerulonephritis
74–5
prevalence 5
prevention/treatment of
diabetic nephropathy
69–73
flow chart 70
primary systemic
vasculitis 84–6, 90
classification 85
prostacyclin 87
prostate-specific antigen
(PSA) 122, 127
prostatic hypertrophy
34, 35, 101
prostatic tumors 125–7
benign 125–6
malignant 126–7
protein:creatinine ratio
8, 15, 78
protein restriction 73
proteinuria 7–9, 11, 15,
35, 41, 44, 45, 46, 59,
64, 66, 74, 75, 78, 80,
94, 95, 100, 128, 130
causes 8
psychosis 18
pulmonary disorders and
SIADH 19
pyelonephritis 100, 102,
105, 106, 107, 111,
131
pyuria 105, 107, 111

quality of life 44, 133,
140

quinolones 102, 105,
107
see also
fluoroquinolones

radical nephrectomy 125
radiological intervention
91
radionucleotide imaging
14
radiotherapy 125, 127
reflux 14
nephropathy 130
renal artery embolism 10
renal artery stenosis/
thrombosis 14, 38, 46,
63, 72, 90, 91
renal biopsy 9, 11, 14,
15, 35, 75, 77, 94, 95,
129
renal bone disease 48,
52–4, 140
contributory factors 53
symptoms 54
treatment 54
renal cell carcinoma
124–5, 126
renal colic 111, 124
renal failure 7, 17, 18,
25, 28, 30, 38, 81,
83, 86, 93, 101, 105,
126
symptoms and signs
42–3
see also acute renal
failure
renal fibrosis 120
renal function in
pregnancy 128
renal function tests 9,
11–12, 14
renal imaging 13–14,
112, 121, 122
renal investigations 7,
9–15
biopsy 15
blood tests 13
function tests 9,
11–12
imaging 13–14
renal pelvic tumors 124,
125, 126
renal perfusion 33, 35

renal replacement
therapy 36, 45, 133–9
conservative care 133
dialysis 133–9
transplantation 139–43
renovascular
lesions/disease 14, 61,
63–4, 90–1
respiratory acidosis and
alkalosis 31
rhabdomyolysis 9, 22,
25, 35, 36, 38
risk factors for
cardiovascular disease
51, 52
for diabetic
nephropathy 69
for kidney stones
109–10
for UTI 98–100
risks of kidney
transplantation 140

salbutamol 26
Salmonella 99, 105
sarcoidosis 87
schistosomiasis 10
sclerosis 87
screening 7
seizures 20, 21, 27, 31
sensors of osmolality 17
sepsis 17, 56, 131, 135
serology 29, 43, 49, 83
serum cystatin
concentration 12, 44
serum electrophoresis 13
serum urea 4, 12, 43
sexual dysfunction 55
sexual intercourse and
UTI 98, 99, 101, 104
sickle-cell disease 10
sirolimus 140, 141
sodium and water
disorders 17–21, 49
hypernatremia 20–1
hyponatremia 17–20
hypo-osmolality 17–20
sodium bicarbonate 22,
37, 38, 46, 55
spironolactone 25
Staphylococcus aureus
99, 105
statins 64

stenting 14, 38, 64, 91, 123, 142
struvite stones 108, 109, 114
subjective global assessment 55
surgery 115–16, 117, 124, 126
  see also transplantation
sweating 18, 20, 22, 23
syndrome of inappropriate secretion of ADH (SIADH) 4, 18
common disorders and 19
diagnostic criteria for 19
systemic disease 83–91
  amyloidosis 89–90
  atherosclerotic renovascular disease 90–1
  cryoglobulinemia 87–8
  HUS 86–7
  lupus erythematosus 83–4
  myeloma 88–9
  primary vasculitis 84–6
  sarcoidosis 87
  sclerosis 87
systemic lupus erythematosus (SLE) 8, 10, 13, 36, 78, 79, 80, 83–4, 88, 90, 130
systemic vasculitis 10

tacrolimus 140, 141
tetany 27, 31
tetracycline as toxin 8
thiazide diuretics 27, 46, 61
thin basement membrane disease 10, 95
thrombosis 14, 34, 135, 140
thrombotic thrombocytopenic purpura (TTP) 4, 86, 87
thyrotoxicosis 28
tissue proteinuria 8

toxic shock syndrome 27
transcellular shifts 23, 25, 26
transitional cell carcinoma 10
transplantation 47, 49, 53, 96, 139–43
  complications 142
  contraindications 139, 140, 143
  problems in pregnancy 130
  risks and benefits 139, 140
  side effects of immunosuppression 141, 143
  survival rates 96, 139
trauma 10, 19, 34, 131
triamterene 25, 109
trimethoprim 102, 105, 106, 124
Trousseau's sign 27, 31
tuberculosis 10, 19, 28
tubular damage 7, 8, 22, 33, 35
tubular disease 10
tubular proteinuria 7, 8
tubulointerstitial nephritis 8, 35, 39, 87
tumors of urinary tract 8, 34, 35, 119, 124–7

UK Prospective Diabetes Study (UKPDS) 71
ultrafiltration 134, 137
ultrasonography 13, 14, 34, 35, 50, 92, 100, 111, 120, 121, 122, 127
urea measurement 9
uremia 34–5, 47, 51, 52, 56
  see also HUS
ureteric disease/obstruction 10, 34
urethritis
  acute 104
  urethral syndrome 104
uric acid stones 108, 109, 115, 119

urinary stasis 128
urinary tract infection (UTI) 4, 7, 9, 10, 93, 98–107, 109, 128
  causes and risk factors 98–100
  obstruction 33
  transplant and 142
  UTI syndromes 101–7
urinary tract obstruction 118–24
  causes 118, 119
  clinical presentation 120, 121
  diagnosis 120–3
  investigation 122
urinary tract tumors 124–7
  kidney 124–5
  prostate 125–7
urine microscopy 7, 9
urine testing 7
US Diabetes Control and Complications Trial (DCCT) 71

vascular complications
  see cardiovascular
vascular disorders 10, 36
ventricular fibrillation 25
verapamil 46
vesicoureteral reflux/obstruction 100, 118, 119
vitamin D deficiency 27, 52–4
volume
  depletion/overload 34, 35, 36, 37, 39, 51, 55, 72
  see also fluid balance
vomiting/nausea 18, 20, 21, 23, 26, 29, 31, 34, 64, 135, 141
von Hippel–Lindau disease 125

Wegener's granulomatosis 84, 85
Wilm's tumor 124, 125